The Smart Woman's Guide to PLASTIC SURGERY

The Smart Woman's Guide to PLASTIC SURGERY

Essential Information from a Female Plastic Surgeon

Jean M. Loftus, M.D.

CB

CONTEMPORARY BOOKS

Library of Congress Cataloging-in-Publication Data

Loftus, Jean M.
    The smart woman's guide to plastic surgery : essential information
from a female plastic surgeon / Jean M. Loftus.
       p.   cm.
    Includes bibliographical reference and index.
    ISBN 0-8092-2583-2
    1. Surgery, Plastic.   2. Face—Surgery.   3. Consumer education.
I. Title.
RD119.L64   1999
617.9'5'082—dc21

617.9508
L827s

99-36975
CIP

Cover photograph of Dr. Jean Loftus by Altman Fleischer,
  Alexander+Altman+Associates, Cincinnati
Interior design by Precision Graphics
Interior illustration by Donna A. Talerico
Interior photographs by Jean M. Loftus, M.D.

Published by Contemporary Books
A division of NTC/Contemporary Publishing Group, Inc.
4255 West Touhy Avenue, Lincolnwood (Chicago), Illinois 60712-1975 U.S.A.
International Standard Book Number: 0-8092-2583-2

00 01 02 03 04 05 VHP 20 19 18 17 16 15 14 13 12 11 10 9 8 7 6 5 4 3 2

For my husband, Jim, whose love, advice, and wisdom
guide my every step

Contents

Foreword

*I*t is with great pleasure that I write a foreword to this book. As a plastic surgeon who has exclusively practiced cosmetic surgery for the past 29 years, I have seen a great number of changes. New techniques have replaced the old. Some operations have been touted and then abandoned in what seemed like a single breath. I have taken part in vigorous debates over which procedures are best and why.

In my career as a cosmetic plastic surgeon, I have learned that among the most important issues is patient safety. *The Smart Woman's Guide to Plastic Surgery* clearly conveys the concepts of plastic surgery with such precision, insight, ethics, and conscience that it is a *must* for any woman considering any type of cosmetic surgery. Both educational and instructional, it provides an excellent basis for the facts about every plastic surgery procedure performed today. In addition to addressing factual concerns, this book explores the emotional aspects of cosmetic surgery and how it affects both you and your family. This book is an indispensable guide that you will want by your side as you journey through the world of cosmetic surgery.

Dr. Jean Loftus sets high standards of honesty and ethics. She places the interest of her patients above all else, and her ideals have been exemplified throughout this book. She has followed a detailed and experienced discussion of the procedures involving the female patient, and perhaps just as importantly, the various concerns that affect all patients, regardless of their gender.

As the art and science of plastic surgery has advanced, we plastic surgeons have learned many things. As we have refined our procedures, we have also come to understand that there is quite another aspect to changing the appearance of our patients. Always careful to discuss what plastic surgery will accomplish, an honest and ethical plastic surgeon also counsels on what it will *not* do.

The Smart Woman's Guide to Plastic Surgery is one more step in the advancement of our profession. It is a clear marker that our frontiers are ever-expanding, but that always foremost in our minds is what we care about most—our patients.

Lawrence B. Robbins, M.D., F.A.C.S
President and Chairman of the Board of Trustees, The American
Society of Aesthetic Plastic Surgery, 1997–1999
Clinical Associate Professor of Plastic and Reconstructive Surgery,
University of Miami School of Medicine

Foreword

*I*n the realm of plastic surgery many factors are important in determining one's satisfaction, but surprisingly none seem as important as the art of listening.

Unfortunately, the patient's ability to listen to and understand her plastic surgeon may be confounded during the preoperative consultation. Her own envisioned appearance may be so vivid that it clouds her ability to see the outcome projected by her plastic surgeon, which may be quite different. Further, she may have such desire for her anticipated operation to go smoothly that she may be blinded to possible risks and drawbacks, as outlined by her surgeon.

The plastic surgeon's understanding of the patient may be no better. He may describe risks in what he considers simple terms, completely unaware that the patient absorbed only a portion of his explanation. He may mistakenly believe that he has clearly described the results that can be reasonably expected and that they are consistent with the goals of the patient, when they are not.

Of course, both make a genuine effort to fully understand one another. Each is undoubtedly doing his or her best, and each assumes they have an understanding. Yet, both are unaware that they are misunderstanding and being misunderstood. Simply put, they are not listening to one another.

To achieve better communication with their surgeon and better understanding of their options, many women seek to educate themselves about plastic surgery. Unfortunately, many obtain their knowledge from the tabloids at the checkout counter of the grocery store. Others read books, magazine articles, and news stories written by laypeople. Although these sources may have honest journalistic intent, they often confuse rather than clarify.

The Smart Woman's Guide to Plastic Surgery provides a clear and balanced view of nearly every plastic surgery procedure. It is honest, straightforward, understandable, and enjoyable to read. Yet, its content is far from elementary.

By separating myths from medical facts, this book covers such practical aspects as the effects of smoking, aspirin, and herbs such as St. John's Wort on surgery and healing. It also addresses controversial issues such as Retin-A, Botox, fat injection, endermologie, and the use of laser therapy. It helps the reader evaluate herself and communicate her desires to her plastic surgeon. It guides the reader in understanding procedures, appreciating limitations, and focusing on her goals. It explains the benefits as well as the drawbacks of each procedure. It examines risks and defines words that are often used by plastic surgeons during the consultation. In short, this book tackles every aspect of plastic surgery.

The text is written clearly and is medically accurate from the beginning chapter on seeking a qualified plastic surgeon to the more complex nuances about breast surgery found in Chapters 7 and 8. I believe that the information provided is not only an excellent resource for potential patients, but is also helpful to doctors in training and plastic surgeons in their first year of practice.

As the Chairman of the Division of Plastic, Reconstructive, and Hand Surgery at the University of Cincinnati, I trained Dr. Loftus and more than 30 other plastic surgeons over the course of 25 years. As a training program director, I work closely with and learn a great deal from and about each plastic surgeon I mentor. Dr. Loftus was one of the more tenacious, insightful, and resilient plastic surgeons that I have had the pleasure of training. She also assumed a unique role as protector and guardian in the care of her patients. She is a focused individual who makes every effort to achieve the high goals she continually sets for herself, and this book represents just one of them.

Dr. Loftus is uniquely suited to author this book. As as woman, she has insight into the minds of other women. As a plastic surgeon, she understands the procedures, their benefits, and their risks, as only a plastic surgeon can. As a writer, she can communicate each concept with unmatched clarity.

Opening this book was the smartest thing you could have done to prepare yourself for your plastic surgery consultation. After reading it, you will better understand your plastic surgeon, and you will facilitate your surgeon's understanding of you. Who knows? You might even listen to one another.

Henry W. Neale, M.D.
Professor and Chairman of the Division of Plastic, Reconstructive,
and Hand Surgery at the University of Cincinnati
Chairman of the American Board of Plastic Surgery, 1995–1996

Acknowledgments

I had assumed that writing a book about something I knew so well would be a simple task. To my humble surprise, I found it was a monumental undertaking. Deciding what I wanted to say was simple, because I say it every day. The difficulty came in developing meaningful explanations that would be easily understood, yet not simplistic. The information then had to be organized so that it would be effortless to follow and enjoyable to read. In order to meet these challenges, I enlisted a number of innocent bystanders who spent much time reviewing the manuscript for accuracy, completeness, understandability, readability, and flow.

My greatest amount of thanks goes to my dear friend Dr. Heidi Murley, who I cannot believe is still my friend after the volumes of manuscript I forced her to edit. Fortunately, Heidi is a general surgeon and is therefore accustomed to debriding refuse and performing colectomies: if Heidi were the punctuation police, she would have arrested me long ago for writing run-on sentences like this one.

Many other thanks are in order, as writing a book is truly a committee project. All have contributed significantly, and they are listed in chronological order of their involvement with the book:

My husband, Dr. James Giffin, for encouraging me to painstakingly make this book the best it could possibly be, for being patient and understanding as I worked on the manuscript, and for providing help with copy and content;

Rick Balkin, the most gentlemanly agent an author could ever hope to have, for accepting this project and representing me in the most professional and attentive manner;

Carol Cartaino, a true doctor's doctor, for immensely improving the manuscript through her insightful ability to see what wasn't there;

Erika Lieberman, my editor at NTC/Contemporary Publishing Group, for recognizing the importance of this work and for providing excellent editorial comments in a gracious style that made refining the manuscript a pleasure;

Julia Anderson, my Senior Project Editor at NTC/Contemporary Publishing Group, for attentively and enthusiastically overseeing the production of this book;

David Stein, my vigilant copyeditor, for his unfailing precision and incredibly high editorial standards;

Kim Bartko, the Art Director at NTC/Contemporary Publishing Group, for ensuring accurate and aesthetic reproductions of the photographs and illustrations;

Dr. David G. Dibbell, Sr., Dr. Henry Neale, Dr. Lawrence Robbins, Dr. Luis Vasconez, and Dr. Ted Lockwood, all renowned plastic surgeons, for scrutinizing the manuscript and providing vital commentary;

Dr. Robin Hardiman, an accomplished plastic surgeon and friend from the trenches, for reviewing the manuscript for completeness and objectivity;

My patients, who shall remain unnamed, for selflessly allowing me to use their stories and photographs for this book (because of their collective generosity, I needed to obtain only three sets of photos from other doctors);

Dr. Edward O. Terino, a world-renowned plastic surgeon for his work with facial implants, for allowing me to use cheek implant photos of one of his patients (with patient consent) in Chapter 6.

Dr. Ted Lockwood, a world-renowned plastic surgeon for developing and refining thigh and body lift procedures, for allowing me to use his patients' photographs (reprinted with permission from *Plastic and Reconstructive Surgery*, 1993, volume 92, number 6, pp. 1112–1122) in Chapter 9;

Coherent Medical Group and Dr. Robert M. Adrian of the Center for Laser Surgery in Washington, D.C., for allowing me to use a set of their photographs in Chapter 12;

Joyce Deloye and Joyce Spencer for their help in typing, retyping, and retyping the manuscript;

Donna Talerico, a freelance artist in Cincinnati, for creating accurate, professional, and aesthetic illustrations before the deadline;

Kathy Jones, the most knowledgeable and skilled plastic surgery nurse anywhere, for filling in details about cosmetic tattooing and skin care;

Beverly Fight, my extraordinary office manager, for contributing indirectly to this book by keeping my life in order while I was writing it;

Dr. David G. Dibbell Sr. and Dr. Henry Neale for lessons in surgery and lessons in life;

Mom and Dad for always encouraging me to reach beyond my potential.

Your Responsibility in Reading This Book

*T*his book does its best to provide you with the most useful, accurate, complete information available about plastic surgery. But techniques and technologies are constantly changing, patients vary in their response to treatments, and the practice of plastic surgery is far more complicated than can be captured in one book.

Realize that this book is intended to facilitate the communication between you and your surgeon—not replace it. If you want advice about cosmetic surgery, you must see a trained medical professional. Do not adopt any of the advice contained in this book without first consulting your physician.

Do not use this book to self-diagnose your problem, prescribe your own treatment, or identify complications. All matters pertaining to your health require medical supervision. Regarding any and all issues related to your preoperative, intraoperative, and postoperative care, you must consult your doctor without hesitation. The author and publisher disclaim any liability arising directly or indirectly from the use of this book.

This Book Is for Women

Men are encouraged to read this book to gain a better understanding of what their female companions are undertaking, but the information contained herein pertains primarily to women. Although some specifics apply to men, many do not. Men have different skin texture, hair patterns, facial features, fat distribution, and body features, all of which merit separate consideration and changes in technique.

Introduction

*A*s a plastic surgeon, I spend much time helping women to understand exactly what they can and cannot expect from cosmetic surgery procedures. I am impressed with the insightful and pointed questions they ask. Most of my patients are intelligent women who simply wish to fight the forces of gravity, change an inherited feature, or look as young as they feel, and they just want to know the facts before choosing to proceed.

The Name of the Game

One question nearly everyone asks is, "What is the difference between 'plastic surgery' and 'cosmetic surgery'?" *Plastic* surgery encompasses both reconstructive surgery and cosmetic surgery. The purpose of *reconstructive* surgery is to restore body form and function for patients who have suffered accidents, cancer, burns, birth defects, hand deformities, or other problems. *Cosmetic* surgery aims solely to improve the appearance of healthy people. It is a sub-specialty of plastic surgery. Thus, all cosmetic surgery is plastic surgery, but not all plastic surgery is cosmetic surgery.

In casual conversation, the more general term "plastic surgery" is used when referring to cosmetic surgery. The public is simply more familiar with this term. For this reason, "plastic surgery" is used in the title of this book. However, this book focuses solely on cosmetic surgery.

Is This Book for You?

Like my patients, you may be eager to have cosmetic surgery. You know it can be safe, and you have seen many good results. But you also know there can be disappointment, frustration, and complications. You seek to educate yourself so that you can decide whether cosmetic surgery is for you. If you do choose to have it, you want to understand exactly what cosmetic surgery can and cannot achieve. And, you understandably want to avoid pitfalls.

Many have told me that nowhere are they able to find objective information about cosmetic surgery. They complain that magazine articles seem polarized toward unbelievable results or horror stories. The books available tend to be superficial and aimed at pitching plastic surgery rather than educating the reader. Even the Internet is cluttered with propaganda. A meaningful book about cosmetic surgery was needed—one that provided complete and unbiased information.

I began writing this book with the goal of teaching the reader about every aspect of cosmetic surgery. Although one book cannot relate every nuance in a field that we surgeons spend a lifetime mastering, much of the information that you, as a consumer, must know is included. This book will arm you with powerful knowledge. This knowledge will help you understand your options and provide you with the balanced view you need to make the right decisions.

The fact that you have in your hands a book on cosmetic surgery is evidence that you do not take this decision lightly. Nor should you. You have chosen to wage war against gravity, age, or genetics so that you may look and feel your best. As with any battle, you may emerge as a winner or a loser, but the more prepared you are, the better you will fare. I wish you the best as you set out on your quest to achieve safe and successful cosmetic surgery, and I believe that you will find this book to be a loyal and expert guide for every step of the way.

The Smart Woman's Guide to PLASTIC SURGERY

Succeeding with Plastic Surgery

Ten Steps for the Best Outcome

*P*lastic surgery permeates Western culture. The mass media love it. It is a favorite topic for talk shows, news segments, and magazine articles. Hollywood loves it. Our favorite actors often show telltale signs of plastic surgery. Advertisers promote it. Local radio stations are infiltrated with ads for cosmetic procedures and the surgeons who allegedly perform them the best. Even you may discuss your aesthetic flaws with your friends or colleagues. Plastic surgery is everywhere. Yet, how much do you really know?

You may have heard that there has been no better time to consider cosmetic surgery. Recent technological developments allow more favorable results than ever before. New techniques such as laser surgery, endoscopic surgery, and Botox injections may provide less invasive alternatives to traditional surgery. The latest implant materials may afford superior results with fewer problems. Pharmaceutical research may provide more effective medications to reduce swelling, bruising, and discomfort. The media gleefully report each new advance. Yet, how much is hype, and how much is real?

Cosmetic surgery has seen an unprecedented explosion in popularity. Between 1996 and 2000 the number of cosmetic procedures more than doubled, growing from one to three million per year in this country alone. This tremendous growth is expected to continue as people of all ages, occupations, and

MARY, *a 22-year-old college student majoring in engineering, was insecure and withdrawn. Even though she had excellent qualifications, her interviews failed to yield job offers. Following surgery to reduce her large nose, her job interviews were more positive, and she soon secured a competitive offer—not because of her appearance, but because of her newfound confidence.*

social classes seek cosmetic surgery. But, despite its popularity, such surgery is not for everyone.

Whether or not cosmetic surgery is for you, only you can decide. This decision will be a complex one. One of your first steps will be to consult with a plastic surgeon, but as you will see, finding a qualified surgeon can be difficult.

The cosmetic surgery boom has made it difficult for prospective patients to identify qualified plastic surgeons. Whereas cosmetic surgery was once performed primarily by plastic surgeons, many other physicians now offer cosmetic procedures. Many physicians, faced with declining insurance reimbursements, have entered the arena of cosmetic surgery, intent to profit from the popularity of this cash-up-front, fee-for-service specialty.

In most states, no law prevents these physicians from advertising as plastic surgeons, even though they may have no formal training in plastic surgery. Even the most sophisticated patients can be fooled. As U.S. Rep. Ron Wyden concluded at a 1989 Congressional hearing, "too many cosmetic surgeons have no formal surgical training. . . . In every state, any medical school graduate with a state license can perform cosmetic surgery. There are no barriers to entry, public or professional."

The search for a qualified plastic surgeon is just one of the obstacles you will face. A carefully planned and organized approach is essential as you pursue a safe and aesthetic result. There are 10 steps that will provide you with what you need to temper your expectations and secure the best outcome.

Step 1: Decide if Plastic Surgery Is Right for You

There are many reasons to consider cosmetic surgery. Many women seek to recapture their youthful appearance. Others desire to improve an inherited trait or to repair sun-damaged skin. Some hope to reverse the effects of pregnancy or weight gain. All have the same final goal: to look and feel their best.

If the decision was easy, this book would not be necessary. The difficulty lies in balancing the potential drawbacks with the anticipated benefits. Cosmetic surgery imposes

Ten Steps for the Best Outcome

1. *Decide if Plastic Surgery Is Right for You*
2. *Find a Qualified Plastic Surgeon*
3. *Evaluate the Surgeon During Your Consultation*
4. *Understand the Risks*
5. *Know the Deleterious Effects of Smoking and Common Medications*
6. *Beware Dangerous Procedures, People, and Information*
7. *Plan Your Surgery*
8. *Pay for It*
9. *Have Your Surgery*
10. *Recover and Resume Your Regular Routine*

TINA, *a 29-year-old manicurist, wanted her breast implants removed. She explained that she had been encouraged by her boyfriend nine years ago to have breast implants placed. Because he paid for the surgery, she had thought there was no reason not to have it. Their relationship dissolved a few years later, but she was left with implants that she never really wanted. She felt self-conscious about her breasts, which seemed to draw a moderate amount of unwanted attention. Had she the option to turn back the clock, she would not have had the implants placed.*

ANN, *a 35-year-old stockbroker, was unable to lose her love handles despite a disciplined diet and rigorous exercise. Following liposuction her result was excellent. Yet, she was disappointed because she still could not fit into her favorite college blue jeans.*

time away from work and play, financial cost, medical risk, and the possibility of disappointment, real or imagined. How can you predict whether your end result will justify braving these obstacles? This book highlights important issues that will play a role in your decision. But, in the end, you alone must decide.

Consult Your Mirror

Physical appearance, inherited and acquired, affects self-image and interactions with others. As long as we have mirrors, our reflections will influence self-esteem. To obtain the most gratifying results from cosmetic surgery, you must first consult your mirror and determine what troubles you. Determine your goals *before* discussing them with your spouse, family, friends, or even your plastic surgeon. Never consider a procedure solely to please another, nor be dissuaded from pursuing a change that you desire (unless your surgeon thinks it is surgically infeasible or medically unsafe). After all, you are the one holding the mirror.

Set Realistic Expectations

The number-one cause of disappointment following cosmetic surgery is failure of the procedure to meet the patient's expectations. Although this is sometimes due to a suboptimal surgical result, it is more often due to unrealistic expectations. Patients may recognize intellectually that there are limits to what they can expect, yet some deny this fact emotionally. Their emotions drive their expectations beyond reality, and they are destined for disappointment.

The best way to protect yourself from unrealistic expectations is through careful discussion with your plastic surgeon. (Because clear communication with your surgeon is essential to success, it is critical that you find one with whom you are comfortable.) Comments such as "Just make me beautiful," are meaningless to your surgeon. Listen carefully when your surgeon mentions limitations in achieving your cosmetic goals, which must be clearly established. Ask questions about all aspects of the outcome you envision and whether it is within reason. The more concrete and specific your expectations, the more likely you are to be satisfied with your final result.

Do not seek plastic surgery with the notion that it will change your life. It will not. Plastic surgery will change your appearance, which may have a powerful impact on your self-perception, but it will not improve relationships, gain new friends, or win back an unfaithful husband. If you have such thoughts, either consciously or subconsciously, cosmetic surgery is almost guaranteed to result in dissatisfaction. Instead of having surgery, openly recognize your expectations and deal with the real problems at hand.

Recognize Asymmetry

You may have noticed that your own photograph does not look exactly like you. This is because you are accustomed to seeing yourself in a mirror, not in a photograph. A photograph represents your true image, which is the opposite of your mirror image. The images are different because we are all asymmetric.

The profound effect of subtle asymmetry can be easily illustrated through photographs of a person that are reversed, split and re-paired left-left and right-right. Because the person is not symmetric, all pictures look different (fig. 1-1).

As with the face, the entire human body is typically asymmetric. Because asymmetries can influence your perception of the final result, your surgeon may point them out to you in advance. (Do not be offended.) Typically a surgeon will ask you to look in a mirror. All mirrors show your face in two dimensions, which enhances abnormalities and asymmetries. This makes them easier to identify and address. To help patients fully appreciate asymmetry, some plastic surgeons use a reverse mirror, which reflects true image rather than mirror image.

Be Wary of Computer Imaging

Computer technology enables plastic surgeons to manipulate patient photographs to demonstrate the effect of a proposed procedure. This may at first seem beneficial because it will help you decide if that procedure is right for you. In reality, computer imaging can be misleading and offer false promises. It shows ideal rather than typical results.

Protect yourself by declining computer imaging until after you have made your decision. Otherwise, even though you will be told that your result is not guaranteed to match the computer-generated "photograph," you will believe your eyes rather than your ears. In any case, seeing a flattering version of yourself may stir your emotions. Remember to keep your expectations in perspective.

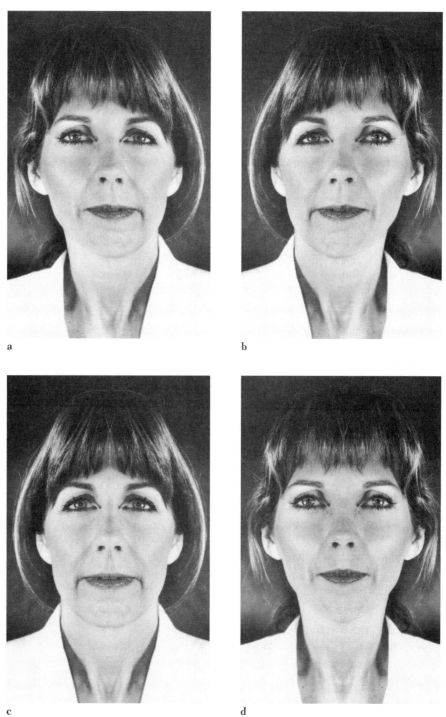

FIGURE 1-1: *(a) Standard photograph. (b) Mirror image of the photo. (c) The left side is matched with the mirror image of the left side. (d) The right side is matched with the mirror image of the right side. All images appear different because this woman, like all of us, is asymmetric.*

Accept the Drawbacks

Anyone who is seriously considering cosmetic surgery must fully appreciate the drawbacks: financial cost, social inconvenience, physical discomfort, and medical risk. (Those issues are detailed later in this book.) Hopefully, *you* are not one of those people who suppresses the objective side of a decision in favor of the emotional side. It is not your style to play down or overlook potential drawbacks. You never say things like, "I'm not worried about discomfort," or "That complication won't happen to me." That's good, because an unwillingness to accept potential complications (however rare) is a sign that one is not ready for cosmetic surgery.

Resolve Inner Conflict

Many people want cosmetic surgery in order to look and feel better, but they are reluctant to accept the medical risk. They want assurance that surgery will be complication-free and that their cosmetic result will be ideal. No plastic surgeons would make such guarantees, and this may create inner conflict for patients. If you find yourself in this situation, do not proceed with surgery until you are able to fully accept the risks.

Another possible source of inner conflict is guilt. Some women have focused their lives on their families, putting their own interests last. This pattern of placing others first becomes ingrained over a lifetime. They may be uneasy about cosmetic surgery, which they perceive as a selfish pursuit. They may feel guilty about spending money on themselves and requiring the attention and patience of family members as they recover. This can be true even when family members are supportive.

Guilt is a common cause of temporary mild depression following cosmetic surgery. If you have a sense of guilt about cosmetic surgery, it is best to address and resolve it *before* proceeding.

A final source of conflict is the well-meaning spouse or significant other. Some partners think they are being supportive by making comments such as, "You look great to me the way you are." These people are completely unaware that such comments are falsely supportive and only compound inner conflict. The message that the woman hears is, "Surgery is completely unnecessary," invalidating her desire to change her appearance. In contrast, a truly sup-

Formula for Success

- *Are you seeking cosmetic surgery for yourself rather than to please another?*

- *Do you have realistic expectations of what the procedure can accomplish?*

- *Do you fully appreciate the drawbacks, such as medical risk, physical discomfort, recovery, and expense?*

- *Have you addressed and resolved inner conflicts?*

- *Does your plastic surgeon understand your goals and agree they are realistic?*

portive comment sounds more like this, "It's your decision. Whatever you decide, I'll back you all the way."

To sum up, if any one ingredient is lacking in the "Formula for Success," then disappointment is likely. But if you can answer "yes" confidently to all the questions listed, then you are likely to be satisfied after cosmetic surgery.

Step 2: Find a Qualified Plastic Surgeon

Finding a qualified plastic surgeon can be challenging. Do not underestimate the complexity of this important task.

Some people assume that if they call their local hospital to ask for a recommendation, they will be referred to the best plastic surgeon at that hospital. On the contrary, telephone referrals are usually divided equally among all plastic surgeons at a hospital, regardless of skill. If you call to ask for a referral, you may simply be given the next name on the list.

One valid way to find a qualified plastic surgeon is by personal recommendation. If a friend was satisfied with the care provided by a surgeon, then chances are that you will be similarly pleased. Or, ask someone in the medical profession, such as your family doctor or a nurse. Keep in mind, however, that doctors and nurses may be familiar only with the physicians at their own hospitals, and they may refer to surgeons based on personality or friendship rather than ability.

Many cosmetic surgery patients prefer not to ask others for recommendations, to preserve the secrecy of their plans. If privacy is important to you, then your task just became more difficult. You may look for a board-certified plastic surgeon in the telephone directories, but, as you will see, deceptive advertising tactics pervade cosmetic surgery. And the problem only starts there.

Board Certification

The American Board of Medical Specialties serves the public interest by overseeing medical boards in the United States. Examples of medical boards include The American Board of Plastic Surgery, The American Board of Anesthesiology, the American Board of Pediatrics, and 21 others. Each board is responsible for certifying only those physicians with the training, judgment, and skill necessary for safe, independent practice within that specialty.

The educated public thinks that it is shrewd to look for the phrase "board certified" as an assurance that their physician is capable and credible. But, the term "board certified" means little, unless the board itself is named. If a cosmetic surgeon states that he or she is board certified, you might assume that it is by the American Board of Plastic Surgery. Yet it could be from any board. Look for physicians who state the exact nature of their certification.

Certification by the American Board of Plastic Surgery

Plastic surgeons who are certified by the American Board of Plastic Surgery (ABPS) must complete all of the following requirements:

- graduate from an accredited medical school,
- complete prerequisite training (typically five years) in an approved surgical residency program,
- complete two to three years of training in an approved plastic surgery training program,
- be recommended by their training program chair for ABPS eligibility,
- pass a comprehensive written examination,
- submit a detailed list of all operations performed during their second year of practice, which is closely scrutinized by the ABPS,
- pass a three-day oral examination, and
- meet moral and ethical standards set forth by the ABPS.

Thus, the term "certified by the American Board of Plastic Surgery" has significant meaning; the term "board certified" means little.

Some doctors who trained in specialties other than plastic and reconstructive surgery do provide high-quality care in cosmetic surgery. In fact, plastic surgeons sometimes invite them to give lectures at plastic surgery meetings.

The American Society of Plastic and Reconstructive Surgeons (ASPRS) inducts only plastic surgeons who are certified by the American Board of Plastic Surgery. To obtain the names of these plastic surgeons in your area, call the ASPRS in Chicago at 800-635-0635 or visit their website at http:\\www.plasticsurgery.org.

SHEILA, a freelance artist and mother of three, decided to give herself a tummy tuck for her 45th birthday. She called a doctor who was listed under "Plastic Surgeons" in the phone book. When she arrived for her appointment, she learned that the doctor was a general practitioner, and not trained to perform a tummy tuck. The office staff assured her that the doctor performed "beautiful" liposuction, as they pointed to a handsome wall certificate attesting to attendance at a weekend mini-course on liposuction. Sheila left the office in frustration and disgust. Determined that this would not happen again, she did research at the library, on the Internet, and over the telephone. She obtained the names of several plastic surgeons certified by the American Board of Plastic Surgery. Following tummy tuck and liposuction of her hips, she was satisfied with her result. Looking back, however, she cannot help but think that she dodged a bullet along the way.

Telephone Directories

In most metropolitan telephone directories, only about two-thirds of the physicians listed under "Plastic and Reconstructive Surgeons" are certified by the American Board of Plastic Surgery (ABPS). Of the remaining third, some may be certified in specialties that, although not limited to plastic surgery, do provide formal training in cosmetic procedures.

Alternatively, some physicians listed may have no formal training at all in cosmetic surgery. Telephone directories in most states do not require physicians to state from which board they received certification. Therefore, physicians may advertise under "Plastic and Reconstructive Surgeons" without being certified by the ABPS or equivalent.

Self-Designated Boards

Furthermore, any physician may seek certification from self-designated boards. A *self-designated* board is not recognized by the American Board of Medical Specialties. Requirements for membership in some of these "boards" are meager. Some self-designated boards have been accused of existing solely to promote their members.

Examples of self-designated boards according to the Board of Medical Specialties:

> The American Board of Aesthetic Plastic Surgeons
> The American Board of Cosmetic Plastic Surgery
> The American Board of Cosmetic Surgery
> The American Board of Cosmetic Breast Surgery
> The American Board of International Cosmetic and Plastic Facial Reconstructive Standards
> The American Board of Laser Surgery
> The American Board of Plastic Esthetic Surgeons

These boards may sound impressive, but according to Joyce D. Nash, author of *What Your Doctor Can't Tell You About Cosmetic Surgery,* "Certification of competency from such organizations is probably meaningless."

Back in 1989, the U.S. House Subcommittee on Regulation held hearings on cosmetic surgery. The Congressional staff report concluded, "Anyone and any group can create a board, call itself anything, and issue certificates suitable for framing. So far, 102 of these self-designated boards have sprung up." Since then, little has changed. Most states have no laws restricting the formation of boards.

Legal but Unqualified Surgeons

The public assumes that if physicians perform a surgical procedure, they are appropriately qualified. This may be true in the hospital setting but is not necessarily true in the doctor's office.

Hospitals are able to ensure quality of care through two mechanisms: privileges and peer review. Physicians must have *privileges* for each procedure they perform. The hospital credentials committee, composed of other physicians, grants permission only to those physicians who are considered qualified to perform a given procedure. Then physicians' performance is subjected to *peer review.* If the quality of care they deliver is deemed substandard, then they may lose their privileges to perform that procedure in the future.

But in the doctor's office, uniform regulations do not exist. In most states, physicians may perform any procedures they choose, whether qualified or not. This unregulated setting has made it possible for untrained physicians to perform cosmetic surgery. If your doctor suggests office surgery, be certain she has privileges to perform the same procedure in the hospital, as evidence that her peers have deemed her qualified. Understand, also, that hospital privileges are neither foolproof nor consistent throughout the country.

To confirm that hospital privileges exist, ask you surgeon at which hospital he or she can perform your procedure. Then call the hospital and ask to speak with someone in the medical staff office. That person should be able to tell you whether your surgeon has privileges for your operation.

Accreditation of Office Surgery Facilities

In an effort to regulate office and freestanding surgical facilities, a few states mandate that they be accredited. Surgical facilities in other states may seek accreditation voluntarily so as to be certain they are providing the best care to their patients.

If your surgeon suggests that your surgery be performed in the office, ask if the office is accredited for surgery and by which organization. The three main organizations for accreditation are:

- The American Association for Accreditation of Ambulatory Surgery Facilities (AAAASF)
- The Accreditation Association for Ambulatory Health Care (AAAHC)
- The Joint Commission on Accreditation of Healthcare Organizations (JCAHO)

Of these, AAAASF is the most common organization for accreditation of plastic surgeons' private surgical facilities. It classes facilities according to their level of anesthesia care. A-rated facilities provide local anesthesia. B-rated facilities provide local and sedation anesthesia. C-rated facilities provide local, sedation, and general anesthesia. The A, B, and C ratings apply only to the AAAASF.

In order to be accreditated, an office surgical facility must meet stringent safety requirements for the layout, equipment, staff, and physicians. Physicians operating at an accredited facility must have privileges to perform the same procedures at an accredited hospital, where peer review applies.

The American Society of Plastic and Reconstructive Surgery (ASPRS) can be contacted to find out which of its members have an accredited surgical facility in your area: 800-635-0635.

Scheduling an Appointment

When calling to schedule your appointment, ask questions freely. Expect the staff to be courteous, informative, and accommodating. If they are not pleasant before surgery, they certainly will not be afterward.

IS THE DOCTOR CERTIFIED BY THE AMERICAN BOARD OF PLASTIC SURGERY (ABPS)?

The receptionist should confirm without hesitation that the doctor is certified by the ABPS or equivalent. If the doctor is not, then the receptionist will invariably explain that the doctor is certified by another board, which is similar in name (see "Self-Designated Boards").

Does ABPS Certification Guarantee That I Will Be Pleased?

No. Many factors determine whether you will be pleased with your result, as explained in Step 1. Further, not every ABPS-certified surgeon is experienced in the procedure you seek. The information and questions provided in each chapter may help you distinguish between those who are experienced and those who hope to gain experience while operating on you.

WHAT IS THE SURGERY FEE?

Although many fees figure into the total price of cosmetic surgery, a telephone quote may only include the surgeon's fee in order to sound more affordable. As the cost of the operating room, anesthesiologist, and implants can add thousands to the total price, you must ask if these are included in the estimate. Do not accept the response "We cannot give you an estimate until we see you." This may be a ploy to lure you into the office.

WHAT IS THE CONSULTATION FEE?

The consultation fee may range from 0 to more than $150. Some plastic surgeons provide free consultations to avoid deterring potential patients. Others charge a fee because they incur an overhead cost with each patient seen in the office. If no consultation fee is charged, then surgical fees may be higher. If you are charged a consultation fee, ask if it can be deducted from your surgical fee.

IS THE DOCTOR PUNCTUAL?

If the receptionist's answer is an unequivocal "yes," then expect to be seen promptly, but be understanding if your surgeon was detained by an operation or an emergency. If you wait more than 30 minutes, it is reasonable to ask the doctor to waive your consultation fee.

Summary Advice

Finding a qualified plastic surgeon may seem like a daunting task. It can be. It's easy to mistakenly conclude that an unqualified physician is a qualified plastic surgeon. Unqualified physicians make great efforts to create the impression that they are plastic surgeons. The term "board certified" is meaningless unless the board is named. In many states, unqualified physicians may legally perform procedures in which they have not been trained. If you understand these issues, then you are well ahead of the general public.

To begin your search, call the ASPRS, ask for the names of surgeons in your area, and carefully evaluate the surgeon during your consultation.

Step 3: Evaluate the Surgeon During Your Consultation

During your consultation, the plastic surgeon should:

- explain each procedure thoroughly, including alternatives, risks, and limitations
- describe recovery in detail
- clearly explain what the proposed procedure will and will not do to improve your appearance, as well as the extent of improvement you can expect
- use understandable terms and answer your questions fully
- put you at ease so that you are comfortable discussing all of your concerns

---

Scheduling an Appointment

A Checklist

☐ *Is the doctor certified by the American Board of Plastic Surgery? (Beware other board certification even if it sounds similar or better.)*

☐ *What is the surgery fee? (Does the cost include the anesthesiologist, the facility, and the implant?)*

☐ *What is the consultation fee? (Is it deducted from the cost of surgery?)*

☐ *Is the doctor punctual? (If so, then expect to be seen promptly.)*

EMILY, a 53-year-old secretary to a high school principal, was tired of looking at her countless spider veins. She saw a plastic surgeon who advertised heavily on television and radio, because she thought he must have substantial experience. Although the surgeon explained the procedure and risks in detail, she did not feel comfortable with him. She had the distinct impression that he would rather have been on the golf course. She knew that treating her leg veins was not major surgery, but she still felt she deserved the full attention of the doctor. Although a second consultation cost her an additional $100, she felt it was well worth it. She was able to establish rapport, and she even looked forward to the procedure.

Evaluating a Plastic Surgeon

A Checklist

☐ *Certified by the American Board of Plastic Surgery?*

☐ *Explained procedures, risks, and alternatives in detail and with clarity?*

☐ *Described recovery time and postoperative care?*

☐ *Conveyed realistic expectations?*

☐ *Answered questions thoroughly?*

☐ *Listened to your concerns?*

☐ *Made you feel comfortable?*

If you achieve this rapport with the first plastic surgeon you see, there is no need to seek another opinion. If not, this does not necessarily mean that the surgeon is a poor one—only that you did not establish rapport. Nevertheless, the surgeon you choose will eventually be operating on you. If you are less than completely comfortable, consider seeing another plastic surgeon. Do not underestimate the importance of rapport.

When you consult with a surgeon, listen for exaggerated claims regarding outcome. If the surgeon promises or guarantees results, be wary. Advertisements may allege that liposuction will result in a 50-pound weight loss or that a face-lift will help you look 20 years younger. Do not be seduced by these extravagant claims, but recognize them as lures to bring you to a particular office and as clues to potentially unethical surgeons.

Questions to Ask During Your Consultation

WILL I BE AWAKE OR ASLEEP DURING SURGERY?

Your surgeon will make a recommendation regarding which type of anesthesia is most appropriate in your case. Do not feel self-conscious or embarrassed if you have concerns about anesthesia, discomfort, or awareness during surgery. These are common concerns, and they should be discussed with your surgeon openly.

ABOUT HOW MANY OF THESE PROCEDURES HAVE YOU PERFORMED IN THE PAST YEAR?

Depending on the surgeon and the operation, the learning curve will vary dramatically. Some surgeons can execute some operations expertly after having performed only a few. Other surgeons continue to improve and refine their techniques after performing it hundreds of times.

The answer will also vary depending on the popularity of the procedure. For common procedures, you may get a specific answer. If you seek a new procedure, do not expect your surgeon to have extensive experience.

How Do You Avoid the Telltale Signs of Surgery?

A *telltale sign* is evidence to others that you have had cosmetic surgery. It is an unnatural physical characteristic that can be attributed to nothing else. Telltale signs are different for each procedure. Examples of telltale signs are a tight face following a face-lift, an unnaturally pale complexion after a phenol chemical peel, and a surprised look after a forehead lift. Some are preventable, whereas others are not. Plastic surgeons should aim to avoid telltale signs when possible. Bring the appropriate list of telltale signs in this book to your consultation, and ask how your surgeon plans to prevent them.

Anesthesia Basics

Three anesthetic techniques are used in cosmetic surgery: general, sedation, and local anesthesia.

General Anesthesia

General anesthesia induces a deep sleep and temporarily paralyzes your body. You will no longer breathe on your own, so the anesthesiologist will place a tube into your trachea. The tube is hooked to a machine that breathes for you. After surgery, you will be awakened, and the tube will be removed. You will feel dazed and tired for the rest of the day. Some people experience nausea following general anesthetic, but with recent improvements in antinausea medications, this is becoming less of a problem.

General anesthesia is needed for large operations such as thigh lift, body lift, tummy tuck, and large-volume liposuction. Many plastic surgeons also prefer it for other operations such as face-lifts, especially when performed in combination with other procedures.

Some patients wonder what would happen if they do not "wake up" following general anesthesia. In truth, this is not a rational concern. Once the anesthetic agents wear off, you will "wake up." General anesthesia is safe, provided you are healthy and that a qualified anesthesiologist or anesthetist is present to administer it and supervise your care.

Sedation Anesthesia

Sedation anesthesia, also called twilight anesthesia or monitored anesthesia care (MAC), uses intravenous medication to induce drowsiness and relaxation. Many procedures, such as face-lift, eyelid surgery, nose surgery, and small-volume liposuction, can be performed comfortably and safely under sedation anesthesia.

Because you continue to breathe on your own, a breathing tube is not necessary. After you are sedated, your surgeon will inject the appropriate area of your body with lidocaine, which is similar to novocaine. Most

Do You Show Pictures of Others Who Have Had the Same Procedure?

The usefulness of viewing before-and-after photos of others who have had the same procedure is overblown. Your surgeon may not show photographs as a matter of policy. Many surgeons do not, because they have found that photographs nourish inflated expectations. You should respect that policy. (The same principles apply here as with computer imaging, described earlier in this chapter.)

If your surgeon suggests that you review photographs of others, be cautious. You will see the best results, even if they are described as average. This

---

likely, you will not feel the injections. Depending on how deeply you are sedated, you may sleep through the entire procedure and remember nothing, or you may wake periodically. If you awaken, you may be aware that you are in the operating room, but most likely will not care. You will feel comfortable, relaxed, and at ease, even if you are prone to anxiety. If you are squeamish about being awake during surgery, make this known to your surgeon or anesthesiologist before your procedure. Thorough discussion with them will likely allay your fears.

Administration of your sedation may be performed by your surgeon or by an anesthesiologist. If administered by your surgeon, your surgeon will be responsible for both performing your surgery and monitoring you during the procedure. This may be too much for one doctor, depending on the technical demands of procedure and the depth of sedation. If administered by an anesthesiologist, your surgeon will be free to concentrate on the procedure while the anesthesiologist keeps you sedated and monitored.

Regarding selection of anesthesia, it is usually safe to follow the recommendation of your surgeon. However, if you are having a lengthy procedure and your surgeon does not recommend an anesthesiologist, you may choose to question that plan.

Local Anesthesia

Local anesthesia involves numbing an area of your body without using sedation beforehand. Injection of local anesthesia, which is similar to novocaine, causes initial mild burning. Burning is soon replaced by numbness. Local anesthesia is appropriate for lip augmentation, removal of moles, and other small procedures.

will heighten your expectations. The fact that another person had excellent results is not a guarantee that you will have even good results. Therefore, protect yourself by declining to look at photographs. Ask instead to see your plastic surgeon's worst results. It is unlikely that you will be allowed to see them, but it lets your surgeon know that you understand the issues pertaining to others' photos. (If you do look at your doctor's recommended photos, the results shown will be the best available, and you should seek another surgeon if they appear unsatisfactory.)

Finally, keep all of this in mind as you look at the photographs in this book. They show generally favorable results. Although your results may be comparable, it is not safe to assume this.

MAY I SPEAK WITH ONE OF YOUR PATIENTS WHO HAS HAD THE SAME PROCEDURE?

In general, this is not a tremendously helpful exercise. No matter what, your experience will be different. For example, you may ask another patient about recovery, but each person's recovery has unique aspects. Also, as with childbirth, she may have forgotten or suppressed the unpleasant aspects of the experience.

If you do speak with another patient, avoid asking if she was pleased she had the procedure performed, as that is no guarantee that you will be satisfied. Avoid asking her about the risks and benefits of the procedure, as laypeople are not qualified to discuss this and may unknowingly give you false information. The most important question is whether the surgeon was available and sensitive to her needs following surgery. (Presumably, the answer will be yes, because your surgeon will refer you only to satisfied patients.)

IN WHICH HOSPITAL DO YOU HAVE PRIVILEGES TO PERFORM THIS PROCEDURE?

Qualified physicians apply for hospital privileges to perform procedures for which they have been properly trained. They welcome the scrutiny of hospital credentials committees and peer review because they are confident of their training and the quality of their care. Physicians with inadequate training will not seek hospital privileges because they will be denied. If your surgeon explains that hospital privileges are unnecessary when the procedure can be performed in the office, be wary.

Before-and-After Photographs

It is standard practice for plastic surgeons to obtain before-and-after photographs. This documents your preoperative appearance and facilitates evaluation of your results.

Your surgeon may show you before-and-after photographs of other patients who have allowed their photos to be viewed. Your surgeon should not allow others to see your photographs without your signed permission.

WILL SURGERY BE PERFORMED IN THE OFFICE OR HOSPITAL?

If you are given the choice, consider the following. Facility charges may not vary much between office and hospital. Office surgery provides privacy, confidentiality, and convenience. Hospital surgery offers a full complement of medical specialists available if you have problems. It also ensures that your surgeon is approved through peer review to perform your procedure. If a lengthy operation such as large-volume liposuction or body lift is planned, you should strongly favor having surgery in the hospital and be concerned if your doctor suggests the office. For most other procedures, you may follow the recommendations of your doctor.

IF SURGERY TAKES LONGER THAN EXPECTED, WHO WILL PAY THE EXTRA COST?

If your procedure is performed in a hospital, then the operating room and anesthesiologist may charge on an hourly basis. Your surgeon must predict the length of your operation to estimate your total fee. If your operation takes longer than expected, then the hospital and anesthesiologist may bill you afterward. Because most cosmetic surgery is paid in advance, an additional bill will be an unpleasant surprise. Clarify this issue with your surgeon prior to surgery.

HOW DO YOU CHARGE FOR REVISION SURGERY?

All surgeons have patients who require revision surgery. The likelihood of needing revision varies with the procedure. Following rhinoplasty or liposuction, 15 to 20 percent of patients seek revision. Following face-lift or eyelid surgery, revision is sought by fewer than 2 percent.

Revision surgery is only appropriate when:

1. the original surgery has left you with asymmetry, deformity, or other problem that both you and your surgeon recognize,
2. the deformity either resulted from or should have been corrected by the original surgery, and
3. the deformity can be improved through further surgery.

Otherwise, surgical revision will not improve your problem.

Surgical revision usually is delayed for 6 to 12 months because changes will continue to occur during this time. Operating too soon can result in overcorrection of the problem. Additionally, many deformities self-correct as they mature, rendering revision unnecessary.

Some surgeons charge a fee for revision that may be as high as the cost of the original operation. Some waive all fees. Others waive only the surgeon's fee, leaving you responsible for the operating room and anesthesia fees. You should understand your surgeon's policy on revision surgery before your original surgery. Most surgeons honor their revision policies for 6 to 12 months, after which time you are responsible for the full cost of revision.

WILL I BE CHARGED FOR FOLLOW-UP APPOINTMENTS?

Following cosmetic surgery, you will require follow-up for suture removal and to ensure you are healing properly without complications. You will see your surgeon once or twice during the week following surgery and once or twice within a month. Anticipate further visits at 3 months, 6 months, and 12 months following some procedures. You should not have to pay for these vis-

During Your Consultation

A Checklist

☐ *Will I be awake or asleep for surgery? (Consider general, sedation, and local anesthesia. Note that you may sleep during either general or sedation anesthesia, although the depth of sleep varies.)*

☐ *About how many of these procedures have you performed in the past year? (The answer may or may not be useful to you.)*

☐ *How do you avoid the telltale signs of surgery? (Bring a list of telltale signs to the doctor's office.)*

☐ *Do you show pictures of others who have had the same procedure? (Remember that most will show you their best pictures.)*

☐ *May I speak with one of your patients who has had the same procedure? (Remember that most will refer you only to their satisfied patients. This is not generally a useful activity.)*

☐ *In which hospital do you have privileges to perform this procedure? (Even if performed in the office, your surgeon should have hospital privileges to perform the procedure as evidence of his qualifications.)*

☐ *Will surgery be performed in the office or hospital? (Consider the advantages of each.)*

☐ *If surgery takes longer than expected, who will pay the extra cost? (When surgery is performed in the hospital, operating room and anesthesia fees may accrue hourly.)*

☐ *How do you charge for revision surgery? (Who pays for the operating room and anesthesia fees? How long does your revision policy apply?)*

☐ *Will I be charged for follow-up appointments? (Expect at least one year of follow-up appointments at no charge.)*

its, as they are a necessary part of your postoperative care. Some surgeons may begin charging you after a year. Others never charge for follow-up appointments. Be sure to understand your surgeon's policy.

Step 4: Understand the Risks

Complications may follow any surgery but are most poorly accepted when they occur after cosmetic surgery. With medically necessary procedures, most complications are outweighed by the operation's need to solve an existing or potential problem. Such a patient is likely to think, "It is unfortunate that I had a complication, but I needed the surgery anyway."

With cosmetic surgery, no existing or potential medical problems have been remedied. Thus, when a complication occurs, a patient is likely to think, "I wish I had never had this procedure done."

But for the best outcome, you must fully acknowledge the risk of complications and be willing to accept any that occur. In addition, if your surgeon is well qualified and experienced, you will have the best chance of having a reasonable outcome following any complication.

The general risks inherent in all procedures are explained below. Specific risks for each procedure will be addressed in subsequent chapters.

Less Improvement than Expected

One of the most common problems is getting less improvement than you expected. All patients should think of this as a potential risk. Although it may be due to inadequate surgery, it is more often due to unrealistic expectations. (Refer to "Set Realistic Expectations" in Step 1 for a full explanation.)

Infection

Infection can occur following any operation and is often treated with antibiotics alone. Occasionally, it is necessary to remove stitches to allow infection to drain. Sometimes the wound is left open, which may result in a more visible scar that can be revised at a later date. If an implant becomes infected, it usually requires removal. For severe infections, additional surgery and admission to the hospital for intravenous antibiotics may be necessary.

Hematoma

A *hematoma* is the accumulation of blood within the surgical site after the skin incision has been closed. A small hematoma usually causes minor bruising and swelling, which may resolve on its own. A large hematoma is more serious. It can threaten the overlying skin, lead to infection, and compromise the final cosmetic result. Surgical exploration and removal of the hematoma is required if it is large.

Seroma

A *seroma* is a collection of clear fluid that weeps into the wound several days following surgery. Your surgeon can remove most seromas with a needle. Surgeons may prevent some seromas by placing plastic drainage tubes at the time of surgery and removing them during a postoperative office visit.

Skin Death or Skin Breakdown

Skin death may occur where skin is under tension or where blood circulation has been compromised. This is often seen following infection or hematoma and is most common in smokers. Treatment involves waiting for the dying skin to separate from the surviving skin. The dead skin is then surgically removed, and the remaining tissue is allowed to heal or is closed surgically. As you might imagine, this may seriously alter the cosmetic outcome.

Asymmetry

A natural and symmetric appearance is the universal goal of patient and surgeon. Surgery, however, may fail to correct pre-existing asymmetry or may create new asymmetry. Mild degrees of asymmetry are normal. Moderate or severe asymmetries may require surgical revision.

Numbness or Tingling

Sensory changes may occur following many operations. Sometimes these changes are expected, such as temporary cheek numbness after a face-lift, persistent abdominal numbness after a tummy tuck, or temporary tingling after liposuction. Other times they are unexpected, such as permanent nipple numbness after breast augmentation. In the majority of instances, sensory changes eventually return to normal. Until that time, they may cause significant distress. Sensory problems are detailed in each chapter.

General Anesthesia

Because general anesthesia involves a greater stress to the body than sedation or local anesthesia, it carries greater risk. Patients who have a history of cardiovascular disease, lung disease, or obesity are at higher risk for complications. Problems can include pneumonia, stroke, heart attack, and blood clots in the legs or lungs. Fortunately these complications are less likely in healthy individuals.

Insurance Coverage for Complications

If you experience a complication from cosmetic surgery, such as infection, pneumonia, or blood clots, you may require hospitalization and further surgery. Most plastic surgeons may not charge you directly, but some may bill your insurance company if you need further surgery. Be certain to clarify this with your surgeon as soon as possible if complications arise. Other doctors, the hospital, and the operating room will definitely charge you.

Your insurance company may not pay for treatment of these medical problems if sustained following cosmetic surgery. (One could argue that this is equivalent to your insurance company denying coverage for treatment of lung cancer because you chose to smoke or for treatment of injuries sustained in an automobile accident because you chose to travel by car. In each scenario, a serious medical problem results from a personal choice.) As hospital-based management of complications can cost tens of thousands of dollars, you should know your company's policy in advance. When you contact your insurance company, ask for a response in writing.

REBECCA, *a 39-year-old convenience store clerk who had successfully lost 80 pounds, thought she was doomed to spend the rest of her life with droopy breasts and a flabby abdomen. When her grandfather left her a small inheritance, she decided to have a breast lift. Although she vowed to quit for one full month prior to surgery, she continued to smoke. But she kept it a secret because she did not want to postpone surgery. Following surgery she had healing problems, and she finally admitted that she had never quit smoking. Her scars were unusually visible. One year later, she desired a tummy tuck. Because complications following tummy tuck in a smoker can be disastrous, she was told she would have to consent to blood testing for nicotine prior to surgery. So far, she has not consented.*

Step 5: Know the Deleterious Effects of Smoking and Common Medications

Smoking

Smoking hinders the body's ability to recover from surgery due to the effect of nicotine. Smokers have a higher rate of infection, skin separation, skin death, and anesthesia complications following certain operations. The difference is so striking that most plastic surgeons insist that patients stop smoking for at least two weeks prior to a face-lift, tummy tuck, or breast lift. Some surgeons may perform surgery despite a patient's continued tobacco use. However, the risks are greater, and the final result may be unsatisfactory. (Nicotine patches and gum must also be discontinued prior to surgery.)

Prescription Medications

If you take prescription medications, advise your surgeon. Some medications may interfere with cosmetic surgery.

Nonprescription Medications and Alcohol

Aspirin, ibuprofen, and similar medications increase the risk of bleeding during surgery and of hematoma following surgery. Many cold and sinus remedies contain hidden aspirin, ibuprofen, or related compounds. Even though a medication may be available without prescription, never assume it is safe. Check with your plastic surgeon.

Avoidance of all nonprescription medications for two weeks prior to surgery should prevent problems. The main exception is plain acetaminophen (Tylenol). It is safe in recommended doses.

VITAMIN E

Vitamin E supplements may contribute to bleeding during and after surgery when taken in doses greater than 200 units per day. They should be discontinued two weeks prior to surgery and may be restarted two to four weeks following surgery.

Vitamin E cream does not contribute to bleeding. It is used by many with the false notion that it facilitates healing and minimizes scarring. It does neither.

HERBAL MEDICATIONS

Some plastic surgeons suspect that herbal medications, such as St. John's Wort, may promote bleeding or other intraoperative problems. Your plastic surgeon may ask you to discontinue all herbal medications prior to surgery and may postpone or cancel your procedure if you do not stop taking them. If you take herbal medications and your doctor does not ask you about them, raise the question yourself.

Nonprescription Medications to Avoid Prior to Surgery

(This list is not exhaustive.)

Advil	Aleve	Anacin	Alka-Seltzer
Anaprox	Ascriptin	Aspirin	Arthritis Pain Formula
Aspergum	Bayer	Bufferin	Congespirin
Dolobid	Ecotrin	Empirin	Dristan Decongestant
Excedrin	Fiorinol	Ibuprofen	Four Way Cold Tablets
Liquiprin	Medipren	Midol 200	Motrin
Nuprin	Pepto-Bismol	Sine-off	Soma Compound

Diet Pills

Redux (dexfenfluramine hydrochloride) and Pondimin (fenfluramine hydrochloride) were voluntarily withdrawn from the market by their manufacturer in 1997, because these diet pills were suspected to cause heart dysfunction in some patients. Meridian, another diet pill, was approved by the FDA in 1998. However, approval by the FDA does not mean that a drug is harmless. Until any drug has been used widely for many years, potentially serious consequences may not be identified.

Fully discuss any past or present diet medications with your plastic surgeon before surgery. This advice applies even if you no longer take diet pills. Some diet pills cause cardiovascular changes that persist long after the pills are discontinued. These changes may predispose you to severe cardiac or pulmonary problems during or after surgery.

Alcohol

Alcohol is a drug that may affect the outcome of your surgery. It may reduce your ability to form clots, increase your bleeding, and heighten your risk of developing a hematoma. To minimize these problems, abstain for at least three days prior to surgery.

Step 6: Beware Dangerous Procedures, People, and Information

No laws govern the procedures that can be performed or by whom they may be performed. In fact, dangerous procedures are performed every day in this country despite medical evidence that they are unsafe. Your awareness of these questionable practices will help you protect yourself.

Fat Injection for Breast Augmentation

Fat injection for the purpose of breast augmentation is dangerous, because injected fat may produce calcium deposits that are seen on breast x-rays. Many breast cancers also attract calcium deposits. A breast x-ray, or mammogram, may not be able to distinguish between benign calcium deposits due to fat injection and those due to breast cancer. This may result in an unnecessary breast biopsy or a delay in diagnosis of breast cancer. Despite well-documented medical evidence that fat injection in the breast is unsafe, it continues to be performed by some physicians. Do not agree to undergo this procedure.

Liquid Silicone Injection

From the 1950s through the early 1980s, liquid silicone was injected into breasts for augmentation. Many women who received those injections later developed deformed, painful, rocklike breasts that have required mastectomy. Hence this procedure is now considered dangerous by most plastic surgeons. Do not consent to the injection of liquid silicone. (Injected liquid silicone differs from silicone gel breast implants. See Chapter 7 for details.)

Nonphysicians

People with no medical training sometimes offer cosmetic makeup tattoos or chemical peels. Approach such offers with caution. Cosmetic tattooing, when performed improperly, may require laser surgery to correct the damage. Chemical peels performed by those without medical training may result in deep facial burns and disfiguring scars. Beware that even minor procedures performed by unqualified individuals can cause permanent damage.

Media Coverage of Cosmetic Surgery

Use caution when considering information on cosmetic surgery provided through television and radio news segments, talk shows, and magazines. The mass media often deliver information in two waves, an initial wave of excitement and inflated expectation, followed by a second wave of disappointment and disaster stories. In the 1980s, the media touted Retin-A as a cure for wrinkles, even though most plastic surgeons noted that its effect was minimal. The subsequent wave exposed Retin-A as ineffective for patients but lucrative for doctors and manufacturers. Similarly, liposuction has been portrayed as a simple, painless procedure that can be performed while the patient is chatting on the telephone with friends. It has also been portrayed as dangerous and ineffective. (Neither portrayal is accurate.)

Step 7: Plan Your Surgery

Planning your operation is similar to planning a trip. You must address many details, and this list will help get you started.

- Consider the time of year. Some procedures are best performed in the cool months. After liposuction, you must wear a compression garment, similar

ELLEN, a 31-year-old advertising assistant, was encouraged by a network news story on stretch marks. The story touted laser removal of stretch marks and explained how simple and effective it was. Ellen was surprised when she learned the truth: lasers do nothing to improve stretch marks. Ellen found it ironic that with her experience in advertising she was easily fooled by these false claims. She had assumed that because the information was presented on a reputable program, it must be true. In the end, she realized that newspeople must sell, too.

to a girdle, continuously for several weeks. This can be cumbersome and uncomfortable in the warm months. After laser resurfacing, you must avoid direct sun exposure for several months, which can be impractical in the summertime.

• If you work weekdays, schedule your operation on a Friday to give you an extra weekend of recovery before returning to your job.

• Expect to have blood drawn at a hospital or lab prior to surgery. A mammogram is usually obtained before breast surgery. If you are over 40 or have medical problems, you may also need an EKG or chest x-ray. Preoperative testing usually requires a separate visit and will take 30 minutes to two hours.

• Purchase two weeks of groceries and household supplies. Prepare single-serving meals and freeze them.

• Anticipate the need following facial surgery to apply iced compresses and elevate your head so as to reduce swelling. Crushed ice can be placed in a plastic bag, wrapped in a small towel, and freshened regularly. Alternatively, a bag of frozen peas is tidy, reusable, and maintains its cold temperature. For elevation of your head, stacked pillows are prone to failure, but you can purchase a dependable backrest in department stores for less than $25. A recliner is a reliable way to elevate your head but may be uncomfortable for sleeping. If you are industrious, you may incline your entire bed by placing cinder blocks under the head posts.

• If you are uncomfortable telling your friends and coworkers you are having cosmetic surgery, then you may wish to tell them
1. you are taking vacation at home
2. you are having reconstructive surgery, which explains why your excuse note is written by a plastic surgeon, or
3. you are having "female surgery."

Few will ask details, especially if you indicate that it is personal.

• Arrange transportation for the day of surgery and for your follow-up appointments. Anticipate that you will not be able to drive on the day of surgery or while you are taking pain medication.

• Ask a friend or family member to stay with you during your first night at home. This person should be willing and able to refresh your ice packs, prepare your food, check on you through the night, recognize problems, and call your doctor. If no one is available, consider hiring a private duty nurse. Your plastic surgeon can direct you to a reputable nursing agency. Anticipate paying $300–$500 per day for this service.

• Fill prescriptions for antibiotics and pain medication prior to the day of surgery. You may pick up the prescriptions from your doctor's office when you pay for your surgery and have them filled when you stock up on groceries. Alternatively, you may have a friend fill them during your operation. You may fill the prescriptions on your way home from surgery, but you will likely prefer to avoid this extra stop.

Step 8: Pay for It

Consider several financial issues before committing to cosmetic surgery. The most obvious concern is whether you can afford it. Then, does the amount spent correlate with the results obtained? Does it make sense to shop around for the best price? What costs are involved? How can cosmetic surgery be financed? Are there circumstances when insurance pays the bills? Each of these topics will be addressed in this section.

> ## Planning Your Surgery
>
> A Checklist
>
> ☐ *Consider the time of year*
>
> ☐ *Schedule your surgery on a Friday if you work weekdays*
>
> ☐ *Expect to have routine preoperative testing*
>
> ☐ *Purchase two weeks of groceries and household supplies*
>
> ☐ *Anticipate the need to reduce swelling following surgery*
>
> ☐ *Decide what to tell your friends and coworkers*
>
> ☐ *Arrange transportation*
>
> ☐ *Ask someone to stay with you your first night at home*
>
> ☐ *Fill your prescriptions prior to surgery*

Cosmetic Surgery Is a Luxury Item

The cost of the cosmetic procedures discussed in this book ranges from $60 to $25,000. At least some procedures are within reach of many people. This explains the rise in popularity of cosmetic procedures among all levels of wage earners. High or low, the cost of cosmetic surgery should be considered in the same light as other luxuries—items you do not need to survive. A trip to the Bahamas, a television set, a fur coat, jewelry, and a candy bar are all examples of luxury items. Although most people can afford inexpensive luxury items, most financial advisors recommend against buying high-end luxury items unless you have sufficient funds available to pay for them. It simply does not make sense to get a face-lift when you are struggling to pay for housing or health insurance.

Justifying the Cost

Some people justify cosmetic surgery by figuring the monthly cost over the time they will have the improvement. For example, the average fee for a facelift is $8,000. Since a face-lift may last 7 to 10 years, the cost can be broken down accordingly: $8,000 divided by 120 months (assuming 10 years) equals $67 per month. The same amount can be spent on monthly facials, which do little to turn back the clock. Similarly, liposuction of the abdomen and hips may cost $6,800 and permanently removes fat cells. The average liposuction patient is 35 years old and can expect to live another 40 years. The cost of liposuction over a lifetime therefore may be $14 per month ($6,800 divided by 480 months). Some people spend more money on their appearance through health club memberships, diet books, medications, and home exercise equipment, yet they remain unable to lose diet-resistant fat. This is not to suggest that liposuction should be performed in lieu of diet and exercise, because the latter clearly offer benefits that liposuction does not. It simply compares the monthly costs of cosmetic surgery and of other things that improve how you look and feel.

Justifying the cost of cosmetic surgery in this way is not necessarily helpful. The best approach is to decide if you have the funds available and whether you want to spend them on cosmetic surgery or another luxury item.

Quality and Price

In the arena of cosmetic surgery, quality and price may correlate, but often do not. The best surgeons may perform quality surgery, develop favorable reputations, and become busy. They then raise prices in response to greater demand. A higher fee, however, does not guarantee a good result. Neither does a lower fee necessarily indicate lesser quality or experience in the realm of cosmetic surgery.

Shopping Around

Shopping around for the best price makes sense when you are purchasing a particular model of a new car, because the car will be the same at every dealer. Such is not the case with plastic surgery. Avoid the mistake of choosing your surgeon based on cost. Rather, find a plastic surgeon who is well trained, who puts you at ease, and who has earned your trust. If you are satisfied with the first plastic surgeon you see, then there is no need to see a second. If you see more than one surgeon, base your decision on quality and rapport, not price.

Fees

Several fees contribute to the overall cost of cosmetic surgery. Be certain you understand which fees are included in your quote for the procedure. An office employee may quote only the surgeon's fee when giving you an estimate. This may not include the anesthesiologist's or the operating room fees. If this is the case, you may believe that the cost of your procedure is much lower than it actually is.

The average fees across the United States for each procedure are itemized in the following chapters. They are based on a survey of plastic surgeons for the year 2000. From 1992 through 2000, cosmetic surgery fees have risen an average of 2 percent per year. Hence, if you are reading this book after the year 2000, factor an additional 2 percent increase in price per year. For example, if you are reading this book in the year 2001, multiply the average price by 1.02; for the year 2002, multiply the average price by 1.04, and so on.

Fees are surprisingly uniform throughout the United States, with the exception of the New York area, where fees are consistently 50 percent higher than the rest of the country.

SURGEON'S FEE

The average surgeon's fee listed in each chapter was derived from a poll of plastic surgeons across the country. You may encounter a surgeon whose fees are outside of the stated range. If your surgeon charges more, you may question whether you will be getting your money's worth. If your surgeon charges less, you should also wonder why.

This fee is applied toward your surgeon's overhead expenses such as employee salaries, rent, and malpractice insurance. After taxes, only about 30 percent of this fee lands in your surgeon's pocket.

ANESTHESIOLOGIST'S FEE

The anesthesiologist's fee usually depends on the length of the procedure. If your surgeon administers your sedation, or if only local anesthesia is used, there should be no anesthesiologist's fee.

FACILITY (OPERATING ROOM) FEE

If surgery is performed in the hospital, there will be a separate operating room fee. If it is performed in the office, there may be a facility fee.

IMPLANT FEE

This fee applies to the cost of medical materials such as breast implants, facial implants, and collagen. The price of your implants may be marked up as little as 10 percent or more than 100 percent. For example, breast implants cost an average of $1,000 per pair from the manufacturer, but you may be charged up to $2,000 for a pair. Your surgeon or the surgery center may profit from the sale of implants.

Financing Your Cosmetic Surgery

Cosmetic surgery, with rare exceptions, is paid in full before surgery. If you lack the liquid assets, you may be able to obtain financing through credit cards or bank cards, payment plans, bank loans, and mortgage plans (which offer the advantage of tax-deductible interest).

But bear in mind that plastic surgery is a luxury item. Few people would borrow money or mortgage their homes to pay for a vacation. So, why consider this for plastic surgery? Think about it.

Insurance Coverage

Cosmetic surgery is not covered by insurance. Exceptions to this rule exist when the surgery corrects a functional problem or deformity. To give some examples, excess upper eyelid skin that interferes with eye opening can be corrected with eyelid surgery. Severely asymmetric breasts can be made symmetric by augmenting the smaller breast with an implant. Paralysis of one side of the face can be improved by a one-sided facelift or forehead lift. A severe hollow of the chin or cheek resulting from trauma or cancer surgery can be restored by placement of an implant or bone graft.

A surgeon who agrees that your anticipated procedure is aimed at improving a deformity or solving a problem may write a letter to your insurance company on your behalf explaining that the surgery should be covered. However, health insurance often will not cover treatment for these medical conditions. (Also, insurance companies may decline coverage for medical complications after cosmetic surgery—see Step 4). Do not rely on coverage from your insurance company, even if you have a legitimate medical need.

Combining with Medically Necessary Operations

If you are in need of a medically indicated procedure and would also like to have a cosmetic procedure, then you may be able to combine them. A common example is combining tummy tuck with hysterectomy. If you would like to pursue this option, discuss it with the surgeon who will perform the medically necessary procedure first. If she agrees that combining operations is appropriate, then she will refer you to a plastic surgeon with whom she has worked. Insurance companies may cover the cost of medically necessary operations, but you will be financially responsible for the portion of fees related to cosmetic surgery. By combining procedures, you may save on the hospital and anesthesia fees.

Step 9: Have Your Surgery

Last-Minute Doubts

You probably will question your decision to have cosmetic surgery countless times before actually proceeding. This is natural. Proceeding with cosmetic surgery takes courage. I did not fully appreciate this until I underwent refractive laser surgery for correction of my vision. I realized that if I was nervous for a painless 15-minute outpatient procedure with a 12-hour recovery, then those undergoing two-hour procedures with one-week recoveries must have serious anxiety. It is natural to have last-minute anxiety and concerns.

Many doubts will race through your mind before surgery. You will be concerned about rational issues such as risk of infection or whether you will be satisfied with your result. You may also be concerned about irrational issues such as whether you will wake up afterward. Central to these concerns is the same basic question: is it worth it? Only you can answer this question. If you feel it is, proceed. If you are uncertain, you should cancel. Because many surgeons charge a fee for canceling within a few days of surgery, ask about this before you cancel. If you are considering cancellation, let your surgeon know as soon as possible.

The Morning of Surgery

Do not eat or drink anything unless otherwise instructed by your surgeon. This may seem like a punitive way to start an already anxious day, but there is a reason. Your stomach must be empty during surgery to minimize the risk of vomiting and make your procedure as safe as possible. If you take prescription medications, ask your doctor whether or not you should take them the morning of surgery with a sip of water. Leave your jewelry at home. Do not drive yourself unless your doctor told you that you would be able to drive home. When you arrive, you will change into a gown. The nurse or anesthesiologist may start an IV and check your vital signs (temperature, blood pressure, heart rate, and respiratory rate). Your surgeon may mark your skin with a felt pen before surgery and may take preoperative photographs. You may be given a sedative before being brought to the operating room.

During Surgery

If you are having general anesthesia, you will remember nothing from the time you are brought to the operating room to the time you wake up in the recovery room. If you are having sedation anesthesia, you will experience deep relaxation or light sleep during surgery, and you will not likely remember details. If you are having local anesthesia, you will be given an injection through a small needle, and you may experience burning followed by numbness. Numbness will last from 2 to 24 hours depending on the agent used. (The differences between general, sedation, and local anesthesia are more fully explained in Step 3.)

Length of Surgery

The length of your procedure may vary greatly depending on your surgeon. Surgeons work at their own pace. A faster surgeon is not more skilled, nor is a slower surgeon doing better work by taking plenty of time. One plastic surgeon I know takes two hours to perform a face-lift, forehead lift, and eyelid surgery. Another surgeon using the same technique takes seven hours. Both surgeons charge the same fee, work in the same setting, and achieve excellent results. Each, however, works at his own pace.

After Surgery

Following most operations, you will be allowed to go home when you are awake and alert. Extensive or uncomfortable procedures, such as tummy tuck, body lift, or large-volume liposuction, usually merit an overnight stay.

Step 10: Recover and Resume Your Regular Routine

This section contains sound advice for the recovering cosmetic surgery patient. Regardless of which procedure you have, revisit this section as the date of your surgery approaches.

The First Few Days

• Expect to look worse before you look better. Nearly all cosmetic surgery procedures involve swelling and bruising. You may even look unsightly temporarily. As swelling and bruising fades, you will begin to see your result.

• If you had surgery on your face or neck, keep your head elevated for two to three days to minimize swelling and speed recovery. Do not underestimate the importance of elevation: it will reduce your recovery time, whereas failure to do so may create disturbing asymmetries.

• Apply an ice pack or iced washcloth to the surgical site. Since swelling peaks at two to three days, application of ice during this period will limit your total swelling. Failure to apply ice following some procedures may result in extensive or prolonged swelling.

• Your doctor will remove your bandages during your first office visit. Stitches will be removed in 3 to 10 days, depending on location. (Absorbable will not require removal.)

• At the end of some procedures, your surgeon may place a drain, which is a small pliable plastic tube connected to a suction reservoir. It evacuates fluid from under your skin and may prevent fluid collections called seromas. Drain removal is performed in the office a few days after surgery and causes brief discomfort.

• Ask your doctor when you may shower, bathe, and wash your hair. Often this is allowed within a day or two of surgery.

• Makeup may be worn 5 to 10 days after facial surgery. Exceptions are carbon dioxide laser resurfacing, phenol peel, and dermabrasion, which require about two weeks without makeup.

• You will be able to return to work between three days and two weeks following most cosmetic operations, depending on the procedure and your occupation.

• Discomfort ranges from minimal following lip augmentation to significant following tummy tuck or body lift. It is also highly variable from person to person. For example, most women find that a face-lift involves minimal discomfort. However, some find that their face-lift was very uncomfortable.

• Do not drive while you are taking pain medication because it will alter your judgment and delay your responses. Following most operations, you will be able to drive once you stop taking pain medication. Exceptions to this rule exist for tummy tuck, thigh lift, and body lift, which require two to four weeks of recovery.

Tips for a Faster Recovery

You may encounter advice from well-meaning friends regarding medications to expedite your recovery. Some remedies have merit, some do not, and some are disputed among plastic surgeons. Always discuss them with your surgeon before taking them.

SUPPLEMENTAL VITAMINS

Except for vitamin E, which in oral doses greater than 200 units per day may promote bleeding, vitamin supplements are considered controversial by many surgeons. Although some surgeons have observed speedier recovery for their patients on vitamin supplements, solid proof is lacking. Some surgeons have found no evidence of speedier recovery and suspect that many supplemental vitamins may even promote bleeding or other problems. They therefore staunchly oppose use of any vitamins around the time of surgery. If you take vitamins, be certain to ask your doctor about them. Do not assume they are harmless.

HERBAL MEDICATIONS

Herbal medications are derived from plants. Examples include gingko biloba, Echinacea, and St. John's Wort. Some herbal medications such as arnica and bromelain may reduce swelling and bruising following surgery. Some plastic surgeons encourage their patients to take these herbs for a more rapid recovery. They are available without prescription, and a five-day course costs $40 to $90.

Because they are derived from plants, many laypeople are drawn to herbal medications and assume that they improve health "naturally" without risk. But some plastic surgeons think herbal medications promote, rather than reduce, bleeding. These surgeons may prohibit them around the time of surgery.

So if you wish to take herbal medications, be certain to have assent from your surgeon.

Out-of-Town Surgery

Some choose to have cosmetic surgery away from where they live because

• *they perceive that results will be better if they travel farther and pay more,*

• *they have heard that the reputation of a particular surgeon is good, or*

• *they seek anonymity.*

Among the problems with seeking surgery away from home, aside from the obvious nuisance and expense of travel, are the very real issues of postoperative care. If you wish to return home immediately after surgery, who will remove your stitches? If you have a complication that becomes evident after you get home, how will your plastic surgeon be able to help you? If your result merits a minor touch-up procedure, will you bother to pursue it if doing so means another trip out of town? These are important drawbacks to consider, especially in light of the fact that, with a little effort, you most likely will be able to find an excellent plastic surgeon close to home.

STEROIDS

Systemic steroids may reduce swelling and provide a psychological lift following surgery. Many doctors give a one-time dose intravenously during surgery; others may have you take oral steroids for a few days. If taken incorrectly, steroids can be dangerous, so they are available through prescription only. If you are a healthy individual with no history of stomach ulcers, it is unlikely that you will have problems. You should discuss steroids with your doctor. (Medical steroids differ from the anabolic steroids taken by athletes to promote muscle growth.)

Back in Public

Most women will be presentable within two weeks of facial surgery, but if you have an important event planned, allow at least three weeks. Following body surgery, you should be presentable in a bathing suit within two to six weeks. However, because everyone heals differently, you may require even more or less time to recover.

Exercise

Exercise, if performed too soon after surgery, may worsen swelling and potentially trigger bleeding. Avoid exercise for two weeks following facial surgery and four weeks following body surgery. Those who have liposuction or submuscular implant placement are particularly prone to swelling with exercise. When you do resume exercise, start with half of your normal routine. Soreness or swelling the following day indicates overexertion. Lack of soreness or swelling indicates that you may gradually increase your workouts.

JANET, *a 25-year-old graduate student in arts administration, felt so well three weeks following submuscular breast augmentation that she went water skiing. She greatly regretted this decision, as the next day she felt horrible. It seemed as though she was starting her recovery period all over again.*

Sexual Relations

Many doctors are uncomfortable discussing sex, and many patients are uncomfortable asking about it. If so, just ask your doctor when you may exercise. In general, as soon as you are allowed to exercise, you may have sex.

Back to the Sun

During the first year following surgery, healing scars may become permanently darkened if exposed to direct sunlight. The same is true for areas of liposuction. Therefore, use extreme caution: protect all surgical sites with potent sun block (SPF 15–40), and completely avoid tanning beds, for one year. (As sun exposure contributes to the problems of aging, *always* avoid the sun without proper protection.)

Scars

Scars are a reality of surgery, and they are permanent. The body heals through scar formation, and the final appearance of your scar depends on several factors. Thin skin, such as the eyelid skin, leaves a barely noticeable scar. In contrast, areas such as the cheek, chest, shoulders, underarms, back, elbows, knees, and buttocks are prone to poor healing and may yield unsightly scars. Skin closed without tension leaves less noticeable scars than skin closed under tension. Most importantly, everyone heals differently. Because of these variables, no one can predict the final appearance of your scar.

In adults, scars are most visible immediately after surgery. Initially they are dark on African-American skin and bright red on Caucasian skin. Early firmness gives way to softening over the course of months. Firm massage of the scar with moisturizing cream may facilitate softening and fading. Start two weeks after surgery and continue twice daily until the scar has faded, which usually takes 3 to 12 months.

Vitamin E is falsely perceived to minimize scar visibility. Whether taken in pill form or as a topical cream, there is no evidence that it improves scar appearance. Some plastic surgeons think it may worsen it.

In summary, your best weapons against visible scars are sun protection, scar massage, and time.

Emotional Recovery

The feelings you may experience following surgery are wide-ranging. Shortly afterward, you may be elated that you had the confidence and courage to undergo surgery. Alternatively, you may become sad or depressed, especially if you develop second thoughts during your recovery period. You may become disappointed or angry if you perceive your result will not be as you expected, even though it may be too early to tell. You may feel guilty that your friends or family members must be called upon to care for you. You may be frustrated and disappointed that others do not notice a change. Often, well-meaning friends will make statements that they consider to be innocuous, such as, "You don't look any different," or "You really did not need the procedure." These statements may aggravate or embarrass you, even though that was not their intent.

Your emotional response in part depends on your psychological preparedness for surgery, your understanding of recovery, and the appropriateness of your expectations. Be aware that despite well-laid plans, your emotions may surprise both you and your family. Interestingly, those who openly share their plans for cosmetic surgery with friends tend to have a smoother emotional recovery than those who try to keep it a secret.

Regardless of your initial response, your emotions will stabilize as your recovery progresses. Most women adjust within days or weeks, although some require months.

Your family's emotional response to your decision to have surgery is another issue. You may have stable emotions but find that your family does not. This seems particularly problematic among teenage children. Teens may strongly express their disapproval before surgery, prompting their mothers to have serious reservations about proceeding. After surgery, they express disgust over their mothers' initial postoperative swelling and bruising, anger over their mothers' discomforts, and criticism of the cosmetic result. You will find that no amount of explaining will help. So deal with them as you would in any matter that primarily concerns you: do what you know to be right, and be patient. With time, they will accept your decision and your new appearance.

LOUISE, a 64-year-old grandmother, underwent laser resurfacing of her face to reduce her wrinkles. The day of surgery, she was elated with her decision to proceed. Two days later, she was in the office for a dressing change and became hysterical when she saw her swollen, crusting, oozing, red face. She was certain she had erred in her decision to have the procedure and wondered out loud whether she would ever see her normal face again. Despite daily office visits and reassurance, she repeatedly broke out into tears. After her skin healed and she was able to see her final result, her emotional instability gave way to genuine pleasure and satisfaction. When she looked at her before-and-after photos, she was overwhelmed by the difference. She apologized profusely for her previous behavior, even though it was not her fault. It is natural to sometimes experience strong emotions following surgery.

Waiting for Your Results

If you are anxious about your appearance following surgery, be patient. Initial results may appear unnatural and unattractive due to swelling and bruising. Although most people see final results between two weeks and two months, the range varies dramatically depending on the patient, the procedure, and the specific technique used. For example, following Botox injections, your final result will be evident within five days. Following rhinoplasty, your nose may continue to change for a year or more. Be patient in judging your final result.

When judging their final result, many women forget the degree of their original problem. Because they forget how differently they looked before

BARBARA, *a 42-year-old soccer mom, expressed disappointment six months following liposuction and a tummy tuck. She felt that surgery did not have much impact on her appearance. In truth, she had a dramatic result, but had forgotten how she looked prior to surgery. When she saw her before-and-after photos compared side by side, she exclaimed, "I didn't look that bad before surgery. Did you switch my pictures with someone else's?" Fortunately, she recognized the underclothing on the before photo, which confirmed that the photos were of her. Some people simply forget—or choose not to remember—their original appearance.*

JOAN, *a 66-year-old widow, planned to have a face-lift, eyelid surgery, and a fore-head lift, but she wanted to keep it a secret. She told her bridge club that she was going to visit relatives for two weeks. Prior to surgery, she bought a new line of makeup with brighter shades and color tones than she previously used. Upon her return, they all commented on how well rested and vibrant she looked and attrib-uted it to her trip and new cosmetics.*

surgery, they may claim that the procedure accomplished nothing. In these cases, a comparison of before-and-after pictures is crucial.

To Tell or Not to Tell?

As the popularity of cosmetic surgery has soared, many people have chosen to be open about their plans for surgery. They have found that their friends and relatives are excited and enthusiastic for them. Some derive confidence from the admiration they receive from others for having the courage to proceed. Yet, not everyone is prepared to be open about their plans for cosmetic surgery, and some prefer to keep it a secret. They want others to notice that they look better, but they do not want them to know why.

We instinctively attribute changes in others' appearance to alteration in hairstyle, clothing, makeup, or weight, but not to surgery. For example, if you had a tummy tuck, your friends may assume you lost weight. So you can simply acknowledge whatever change your friends perceive and thank them for noticing. Furthermore, you can change your hairstyle or color and buy a few new outfits. This will provide others with a concrete reason for your new look.

In mid-1993, a well-known public figure appeared to have had excellent cosmetic surgery for facial rejuvenation. Interestingly, this went unnoticed by the media because of a concurrent change in her hairstyle, clothing, and makeup. If someone in the national public eye can keep cosmetic surgery a secret, so can you. It's your choice.

2

Trading Faces

Face-Lift

*I*f you are reading this chapter, you are probably over 40 and frustrated that you appear older than you feel. Each time you look in the mirror, you catch glimpses of your mother. The skin of your cheeks has fallen, and you have developed heavy skin folds around your nose and mouth. Your neck has lost its distinction from your jawline. You may be ready for a face-lift, but how can you be sure?

BARBARA, *a 51-year-old empty nester, wanted to rejoin the work-force at the managerial level. Despite her enthusiasm and experience, she had difficulty finding the right opportunity. The reason, she suspected, was her mature appearance. A face-lift subtracted several years from her apparent age and bolstered her self-confidence. She received three attractive job offers. She later appropriately concluded that the offers came because of her improved self-esteem, not because of her actual appearance.*

The Good News: Things a Face-Lift Can Improve

The soft tissues of your cheek and neck descend due to aging and gravity. A face-lift will counter this by removing excess skin and tightening the remaining tissues.

Sagging Cheeks

Study your face in the mirror. You may see a heavy skin fold, the *nasolabial fold,* around either side of your nose and mouth. You may see that your once-smooth jawline has been replaced by jowls.

If you place your fingers on the center of your check and press the skin up and back, you will see the effects of a face-lift (fig. 2-1). Your heavy skin

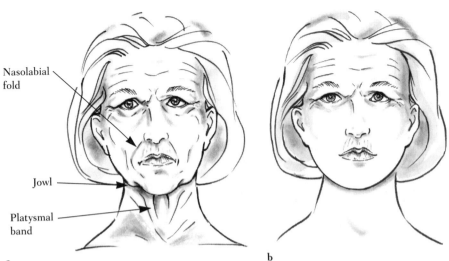

Nasolabial
fold

Jowl

Platysmal
band

a   **b**

FIGURE 2-1: *The effects of a face-lift. (a) Features of an aging face. (b) After a face-lift the jowls
and nasolabial folds (around the mouth) are improved and the neck appears tighter and
smoother. The forehead, eyes, and lips are unchanged.*

folds are lifted and improved, but they will not disappear. Your jowls may be
eliminated. If this maneuver improves the appearance of your cheeks and
jawline to your satisfaction, then you may be ready for a face-lift.

To see how much skin can be removed, use your thumb and forefinger to
gently pinch the skin in front of your ear. The amount you can pinch is the
amount that can be removed during your face-lift.

Sagging Neck

To assess your neck, you must be able to see your profile without turning your
head. This can be accomplished by using two mirrors. Stand with one shoulder toward a wall mirror. Hold a small mirror in front of you, in your opposite
hand. As you look straight ahead into the small mirror, slowly tilt it toward
the wall mirror until your facial profile comes into view. As you study your
profile, you may notice a few undesirable features.

The once-sharp angle between your jawline and neck may have given way
to a blunt angle with loss of definition. In other words, it may no longer be
evident where your jawline ends and your neck begins (fig. 2-2).

One of your neck muscles, the *platysma*, may have formed bands that are
prominent on either side of your midline. In severe cases, you may develop a
"turkey gobbler," which is so called because it resembles the wattle of a

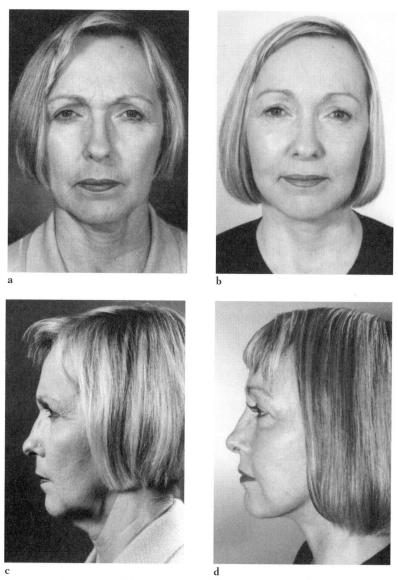

(a and c) Before face-lift. (b and d) After face-lift. This woman also had a forehead lift and eyelid surgery. This combination is far more common than face-lift alone. Note that the jowls are gone, the nasolabial folds are improved, and the "turkey-gobbler" neck has been eliminated.

turkey. It may be thick or thin and is due to prominence of the platysma, sagginess of the neck skin, and accumulation of fat.

Another neck problem, due to fat alone, is the double chin.

Sagging neck, turkey-gobbler appearance, and double chin are all corrected by a face-lift. To see the effect of a face-lift on your neck, place your

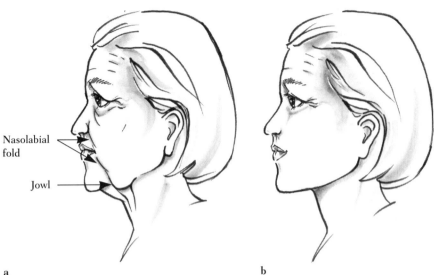

Nasolabial fold

Jowl

a   b

FIGURE 2-2: *The effects of a face-lift. (a) Profile of an aging face. (b) After a face-lift the jowls are gone and the "turkey-gobbler" neck has been refined, but the forehead and eyes are unchanged.*

fingers on both sides of your neck and gently stretch your skin backward and upward. If you like what you see, you will likely be satisfied with the results of a face-lift.

The Bad News: Things a Face-Lift Cannot Improve

A face-lift can have a dramatic impact on appearance, but it will not solve all the problems of an aging face.

Forehead and Eyelids

A face-lift will only lift your lower face and neck. It will not change the appearance of your forehead or eyelids. Therefore, a face-lift alone may create facial disharmony, as your rejuvenated cheeks and neck may cause your forehead and eyes to appear older by comparison. To obtain a uniformly youthful appearance, many

MARY, *a 67-year-old grandmother, cherished her 3-year-old grandson. However, when he sat on her lap, he would play with her "turkey gobbler" neck. Faced with the choices of enduring the embarrassment, avoiding her grandchild, or fixing her neck, she chose the last.*

SANDRA, *a 67-year-old retired college professor, had a face-lift and neck lift without forehead lift or eyelid surgery. She was pleased with her lower face and neck but disappointed that her upper face still looked many years older. Within three months, she proceeded with a forehead lift and eyelid surgery. Although in the end she was satisfied with her appearance, she wished she had undergone all procedures at the beginning.*

women opt for face-lift, forehead lift, and eyelid surgery at the same time.

Wrinkles and Skin Problems

A face-lift will not affect the quality of your skin. Therefore, wrinkles, texture problems, and color irregularities will not be improved. Laser resurfacing, chemical peel, and dermabrasion complement a face-lift because they address these problems.

On your cheeks, chin, or neck, these additional procedures are best delayed until three months after a face-lift, when the healing process has restored full circulation to the skin. But on your forehead, lips, nose, and crow's feet, they may be safely performed on the day of your face-lift because the circulation to these areas is not affected by a face-lift.

When to Start Thinking About a Face-Lift

Women as young as 30 or as old as 85 seek this procedure. The most common age for a first face-lift is 45–60 years, but appearance, not age, is the main factor. The aging process does not take place at a fixed rate. Accelerated aging may occur in response to illness, emotional stress, depression, tobacco use, and, of course, heavy sun exposure. When considering the timing for a face-lift for yourself, perform the maneuvers described previously. If you are satisfied with the improvement you see, then it is time to start thinking about a face-lift.

Face-Lift Techniques

As with many procedures in plastic surgery, there is more than one way to accomplish a good face-lift. Years of spirited debate and volumes of published material have not led plastic surgeons to a consensus regarding which face-lift technique is the best.

A face-lift is the result of the artistry, judgment, and skill of your surgeon. We surgeons select the technique that produces the best and most reliable results in our own hands. Perhaps here, more than anywhere else in plastic

---

BETTY, *a 53-year-old intensive care nurse, survived a stormy divorce only to discover a new set of problems. Although she was eager to meet men, she had not been on a date in almost 30 years and found that she was surprisingly self-conscious about her age. Following a face-lift, eyelid surgery, and a forehead lift, she felt better about herself and dating. Her most satisfying moment came when she saw her ex-husband at a social gathering. Although they did not speak, she caught his glimpse from across the room. The expression on his face clearly said, "Wow, I can't believe how good you look!" She defiantly returned the unspoken message, "Yes, I do . . . and I've gotten over you."*

PAT, *a 50-year-old Realtor, had a face-lift, forehead lift, and eyelid surgery. Although she was pleased with her more youthful appearance, she was disappointed with the persistent crow's feet around her eyes and the wrinkles around her lips. She complained that she had "old skin on a young face." Botox treatments, skin care, and micro peels—all minor procedures with immediate recovery—improved her wrinkles, softened her skin, and enhanced her overall appearance (see Chapter 11).*

surgery, knowing someone who has had successful results can be essential in helping you choose a surgeon.

If you are uncomfortable with the recommended technique, with the explanation of its rationale, or with the answers to your questions, then seek a second opinion.

Components of a Face-Lift

Most face-lift techniques have five basic parts.

Face
- Removing excess facial skin
- Tightening tissue under the skin

Neck
- Removing excess neck skin
- Tightening the neck muscle
- Removing neck fat

Each part can be modified and combined with other parts in a variety of ways to achieve your goals. Not all parts are necessary in every case.

Of the five parts listed above, three are aimed at improving the neck. So when you seek a face-lift, expect your neck to be included. Be certain you understand exactly how your surgeon defines a face-lift before you proceed. Some surgeons divide a "face-lift" into two procedures, on the face and on the neck, each with separate charges. If so, the total cost should not be significantly more than if they were performed together.

Skin-Only Face-Lift

The *skin-only* face-lift, also known as a *one-layer* face-lift, involves removal of excess skin of the face and neck, with no surgery on the deeper tissues. This technique may be appropriate in some instances; however, some plastic surgeons hold that it is less effective than the two-layer technique, and it may not last as long.

The Two-Layer (SMAS) Face-Lift

The two-layer technique is one of the most common. The first layer is facial and neck skin, the excess of which is removed. The second layer is tissue under the skin, which is lifted or tightened. The layer under the facial skin is a fibrous tissue similar to the gristle on a steak, only much thinner and lighter. It is called the SMAS (subcutaneous musculo-aponeurotic substance) and is located only on the face. In the neck, the second layer is a thin, broad muscle called the platysma. With the two-layer technique, both the SMAS and platysma are tightened. Multiple techniques are available for tightening the SMAS, and plastic surgeons vigorously debate which one is best.

The two-layer approach allows surgeons to tighten and lift each layer independently. We tighten the SMAS and platysma snugly, to improve jowls, heavy folds around the mouth, and turkey-gobbler neck. Then we drape the skin of the face and neck over this layer to achieve a natural appearance without tension. This combination provides a significant lift, but without the associated tight or windblown look that can develop when the skin alone is overly tightened.

A final benefit of the two-layer technique is potential cheek augmentation. Some women with flat cheekbones seek more cheek projection. Cheek augmentation typically involves placement of implants on top of your cheekbones (see Chapter 6). However, if you are having a two-layer face-lift, your surgeon may instead use your extra SMAS to build up your cheeks.

Subperiosteal (Deep) Face-Lift

Although the title of this chapter is "Trading Faces," the last thing you want from a face-lift is to look like a different person. The *deep* face-lift, also called *subperiosteal* face-lift, may do just that. With this technique, all tissues, including the SMAS and facial muscles, are separated from the underlying bone and lifted higher. The technique can cause persistent swelling, result in droopy lower eyelids, and alter basic facial characteristics.

A face-lift that turns back the clock to a younger you is enthusiastically received, but one that alters facial characteristics poses problems. By the age of 40 or 50, your perception of yourself is so entrenched that any change in basic facial structure, no matter how good, makes for a difficult adjustment. The older you are, the harder it will be for you to adapt to a new look following a subperiosteal lift.

Some plastic surgeons report favorable experience with subperiosteal face-lifts. If your surgeon recommends this technique, this is an appropriate situation in which to ask to speak with a previous patient. You may also ask to look at before-and-after photos and inspect them for any alterations in basic appearance.

Cheek Lift

The *cheek* lift, also called a mid-face-lift, evolved in the mid-1990s. Many surgeons have adapted this procedure

JACKIE, *a 53-year-old attorney, wanted a face-lift, but she did not want to have the problems of her best friend's subperiosteal face-lift. Although her friend appeared more youthful, the swelling persisted for 10 weeks. Jackie also thought her friend simply looked different. It was hard for Jackie to point to the change, but she said, "It is as though she now looks like her sister, except that she has no sisters." Jackie wanted neither a long recovery period nor to look like a different person. She had a SMAS face-lift, her swelling improved in two weeks, and she looked like a younger version of herself.*

because of its effectiveness in rejuvenating the cheek area. It is a limited version of the subperiosteal lift, and, not surprisingly, it poses the same potential problems. It may alter your basic appearance, cause droopy lower eyelids, and leave you swollen for weeks or months. Its long-term effects are not yet known. If your surgeon proposes this procedure, ask about risks, alternatives, how many she or he has performed, and the reasons for recommending it to you.

Mini Face-Lift

A *mini* face-lift usually employs standard face-lift incisions but involves very limited surgery under the skin. When you hear "mini face-lift," you should think of the word "minimal." Most mini face-lifts involve minimal surgery, remove minimal skin, and provide minimal improvement. If your surgeon suggests a mini face-lift, you may wish to question the plan or seek a second opinion. Often, those who are advised to have a mini face-lift do not need a face-lift at all.

Neck-Only Lift

A *neck-only* lift, also called platysma-plasty, is for those who have a sagging platysma muscle without a sagging face and without excess neck skin—an uncommon combination. The surgeon makes a small incision under the chin, tightens the platysma muscle, and, if needed, removes neck fat.

If you pursue this procedure, you must limit your expectations. Neck-only lifts performed through a single incision under the chin are unable to remove excess skin and will not provide the same degree of improvement as a full face and neck lift, in which neck skin is tightened. Hence this operation is rarely performed.

Endoscopic Face-Lift

The *endoscopic* face-lift may seem appealing because the endoscope allows surgery through small incisions. This technique may be appropriate for young people with early jowls and no loose skin—a rare combination. Most face-lift candidates, however, have excess skin, the removal of which mandates long incisions. This voids the benefit of an endoscopic technique.

Laser Face-Lift

Laser face-lift is no different than conventional face-lift except that the dissection portion of the operation is performed with a different instrument, the laser. The final result is no better and lasts no longer than the results of a conventional face-lift. Use of the laser may increase your cost by several hundred dollars. Most plastic surgeons consider the use of laser unjustified as it fails to provide a clear benefit.

Incisions and Scars

All face-lift techniques require an incision that extends from above your ear, down the front of your ear, around your ear lobe, up the back of your ear, and into your hairline behind your ear. There is another incision beneath your chin (fig. 2-3). Most scars from a face-lift are hard to see once they heal. Your scars should fade beyond detection in 4 to 12 weeks, except for the scar behind your ear, which may become wide and thick. Two weeks after surgery, they may be concealed with makeup.

There are exceptions. If your incision heals poorly or is placed in a visible area such as below your hairline, your scars may be noticeable. Ask your surgeon to show you where your incisions will be.

What to Expect

Face-lifts are commonly performed under sedation anesthesia. Most surgeons recommend that you stay overnight so that nurses can keep cold compresses on your face, keep your head elevated, and observe you for complications. Discomfort is mild and will be controlled with acetaminophen

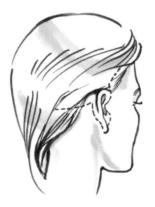
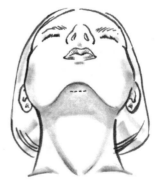

a   b

FIGURE 2-3: *Face-lift incisions. The incisions for a face-lift are well hidden (a) behind the hairline, around the ear, and (b) under the chin.*

(Tylenol) or a mild prescription pain medication. Following most face-lift techniques, you will be presentable in public in two weeks, and your final result will be evident in four to eight weeks.

To help you plan for and recover from your procedure, re-read Steps 7 and 10 of Chapter 1.

Vital Statistics

Anesthesia: Sedation or general.

Location of operation: Office or hospital.

Length of surgery: 2–4 hours. If you are also having eyelid surgery and forehead lift, the total time may be 3–6 hours.

Length of stay: An overnight stay may be recommended to monitor for hematoma (blood collection under your skin) and to ensure that you sleep with your head elevated.

Discomfort: Mild. Anticipate 0–3 days of pain medication; Tylenol alone may be adequate. Many women report no discomfort afterward. If you have pain, contact your surgeon immediately to be certain you do not have a hematoma.

Swelling and bruising: Improve in 2 weeks, but will last longer after deep (subperiosteal) face-lift. Your face will feel tight for the first few weeks due to swelling. You can reduce swelling through constant head elevation and frequent application of cold compresses.

Numbness: Cheek numbness lasts several weeks.

Bandages: Changed in 1–2 days.

Stitches: Removed in 4–10 days (4–6 days for ears and chin, 7–10 days for hairline). Staples may be used behind your hairline. Neither stitch nor staple removal is painful.

Drain: If your surgeon places a drain at the time of surgery, it will be removed in 1–2 days.

Makeup: May be worn in 1–2 weeks.

Presentable in public: You should be presentable within 2 weeks with the help of makeup. To be certain, allow 3 weeks before an important event. If a deep (subperiosteal) lift is planned, allow 1–2 months because swelling will be greater.

Work: You may feel capable of returning within 5 days, but your appearance will be the limiting factor.

Exercise: May be resumed in 2–3 weeks.

Sun protection: 6 months with SPF 15 or higher.

Final result: Seen in 4–8 weeks following most face-lifts, but 2–4 months following deep (subperiosteal) face-lift because swelling is worse.

Complications

When your operation is performed by a qualified plastic surgeon, both your procedure and recovery will likely be uneventful. Even in ideal circumstances, however, complications may occur. In addition to the specific complications mentioned here, refer to Chapter 1 for general complications with any procedure.

Hematoma

A hematoma is a collection of blood that may form under the skin, usually within a day of surgery. If a large hematoma is untreated, the skin over it may die (see "Skin Death").

Hematomas are suspected when patients develop one-sided facial pain following face-lift. If you have such pain, notify your doctor immediately. A small hematoma may be removed without re-opening the incision. If you have a medium or a large hematoma, your surgeon will probably bring you back to the operating room immediately to remove the hematoma through your original incision. If treated soon enough, even large hematomas will not affect your final results.

The average risk of hematoma is 3 to 4 percent, and this risk may be higher in redheads due to their skin's rich circulation. Hematoma is also more common in those with high blood pressure and those taking aspirin, ibuprofen, or other medications that interfere with blood clotting. Therefore, stop all aspirin products two weeks before surgery and stop ibuprofen three days prior to surgery. If you take any prescription arthritis medication, notify your doctor. (Acetaminophen, which does not interfere with blood clotting, may be taken up to the time of surgery.)

Skin Death

Skin death can occur in front of or behind your ear. It may result in a large wound that can take several weeks to heal. During that time, the wound is bandaged and expected to heal on its own. The healed wound leaves a thick, irregular, and highly visible scar.

Skin death occurs most often when the patient has an untreated hematoma or smokes. Both factors reduce circulation to the skin. Therefore, hematomas

---

When Can I Stop Worrying About Complications?

Most complications occur within a predictable time following surgery. If you do not develop them within the time periods noted, you can fairly conclude that you are probably free of these complications:

Time Since Surgery	Possible Complication
2 days	Hematoma
1 day	Facial weakness
1 day	Ear numbness
2 weeks	Skin death
2 weeks	Infection
6 months	Early relapse

should be treated immediately, and smokers should quit smoking long before surgery. Many plastic surgeons deny face-lifts to active smokers. Smokers who quit before surgery remain at higher risk for skin death than those who never smoked, but they are at lower risk than those who continue smoking.

Facial Weakness or Paralysis

Facial weakness may be temporary or permanent. It is caused by injury to the facial nerve or one of its branches that control facial expression. Injury may occur to these nerves if they are cut, stretched, or cauterized* during surgery. This may lead to loss of one or more facial expressions: raising the eyebrows, scowling, closing the eyes, squinting, smiling, frowning, and pursing the lips.

Full facial expression generally returns within three months, because most nerve injuries are due to stretching or cauterization, which are temporary insults. But if a nerve is cut, function may not return. You may permanently be left with a droopy eyebrow, an inability to close your eye, an immobile cheek, or a droopy mouth, depending upon which branch was injured. These deficiencies are made obvious by comparison to the normal opposite side. This poses a major cosmetic problem and further surgery may be sought to improve symmetry. Alternatively, Botox, an agent that causes temporary muscle weakness, may be injected into the unaffected side to lessen asymmetry. Fortunately, the risk of permanent facial weakness or paralysis is less than 1 percent.

GERALDINE, *a 63-year-old nightclub owner, was so ashamed of smoking that she did not report it before surgery. She felt certain she could quit before her face-lift, but as surgery approached, she simply could not stop smoking. Faced with the embarrassment of confessing her habit, she chose instead to remain silent. After all, how much harm could a few cigarettes cause? She discovered the answer shortly after surgery when a small patch of skin died in front of one ear and behind both ears. Fortunately, she is now able to conceal the resultant scars with makeup and a change in hairstyle. Although she regrets having smoked before her face-lift, she is grateful that this experience provided her with the incentive she needed to quit smoking.*

Infection

Because of the excellent circulation to the face, the risk of infection is less than 1 percent. However, if infection does occur, it may be devastating and cause skin death, open wounds, and unsightly scars.

Ear Numbness

Whereas transient cheek numbness following face-lift is expected, numbness of the ear is not. Temporary numbness of the skin surrounding the ear

---

Surgical disruption of small blood vessels can cause bleeding. To stop the bleeding, your surgeon may cauterize the bleeding vessel—using an instrument that delivers a low-level electrical current to it. Nearby nerves may be temporarily injured, resulting in weakness or paralysis.

may be caused by surgical injury of the great auricular nerve. Permanent numbness can result if that nerve was cut. Damage to the great auricular nerve is rare, occurring in fewer than 1 percent of patients. If a cut nerve is recognized during surgery, it can be repaired. Subsequent recovery of sensation may be partial, complete, or confounded by sharp pains in the neck or ear.

Early Relapse

Early relapse is the premature return of sagging skin and jowls, well before the 7 to 10 years a face-lift is expected to last. Relapse may occur within six months. The cause of relapse is not clear, but it seems to be more common in women with fair complexions and sun-damaged skin. Early relapse occurs in 1 percent and can be treated by another face-lift, which is usually more lasting.

Telltale Signs

Prior to surgery, ask how your surgeon plans to prevent each of the following telltale signs of cosmetic surgery (see "Questions to Ask" at the end of this chapter).

Attached Earlobe

An attached earlobe, "pixie ear," occurs when too much skin has been removed nearby. The remaining, stretched skin pulls the earlobe down and into the surrounding skin (fig. 2-4). It can be corrected through minor surgery.

Open Ear Canal

A wide-open ear canal appears unnatural. Look at the side of your head by using two mirrors. (To do this, stand with your shoulder to a wall mirror. Hold a hand mirror in front of you and tilt it toward the wall mirror. As you look straight ahead into the hand mirror, you should see the reflection of your profile in it.) Notice that the cartilage in front of your ear canal partially hides your canal from view. If a face-lift places tension on the skin of this cartilage, it will be pulled forward and widen your ear canal (fig. 2-4).

Most people do not notice a wide-open ear canal and are not bothered by it. At any rate, it is difficult to fix until your facial skin is loose. If you wish to have it fixed, you may need to wait for your next face-lift.

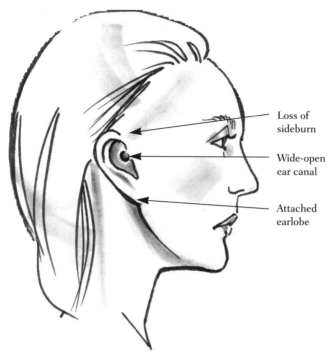

Loss of
sideburn

Wide-open
ear canal

Attached
earlobe

FIGURE 2-4: *Telltale signs of a face-lift. Possible telltale signs following a face-lift include attached earlobe, wide-open ear canal, tight face, and absent sideburn. (Your surgeon will try to avoid telltale signs.)*

Tight Face

A tightly pulled face, also called the "wind-tunnel look," appears unnatural and results from removing too much skin. It can also develop following multiple face-lifts. Once skin has been removed, it cannot be easily replaced. Thus, a tight face is difficult to correct.

Loss of Sideburns

Your sideburns will migrate upward with each face-lift. After two face-lifts, your sideburns can be lost entirely. Many women do not consider sideburns a vital facial feature but soon realize their importance if they are lost (fig. 2-4). A modification in surgical technique may preserve your sideburns. High or absent sideburns are difficult to correct.

Visible Scar

The scar in front of your ear usually fades and becomes imperceptible within 4 to 12 weeks. This is particularly true if the incision zigzags with the contour of your ear (fig. 2-3a). If, however, the incision in front of your ear is a straight line, it may be more visible.

The skin behind your ear may sometimes widen and yield an unsightly scar. Fortunately, this is hidden by your ear and your hair (fig. 2-3a). An obvious scar is preventable by planning your incision into the hair rather than below it. If, however, the incision behind your ear is made below your hairline, this scar may be highly visible, especially if you wear your hair up. A wide scar below the hairline is difficult to correct surgically and is hidden only through hairstyle modification. Women who have short hair or wear their hair up have greater difficulty concealing this telltale sign.

Even if the scar is planned ideally, it may be visible behind your ear before it goes into the hairline. Again, modifications in hair style should help conceal this.

Skin Irregularities and Cobblestone Appearance

Fat is a natural buffer between skin and muscle. An unnatural cobblestone appearance can result if your surgeon removes too much face or neck fat.

Cost

In the United States, the range of total fees for a face-lift extends from $6,000 to $10,000. The average cost is:

Surgeon's fee	$5,000
Anesthesiologist's fee	$1,000
Operating room (facility) fee	$1,500
Hospital fee for overnight stay	$ 500
Total	$8,000

See "Fees" in Chapter 1 for various factors that might affect your own actual cost.

Duration of Results

A face-lift may reduce your apparent age by a decade, but the aging process does not stop. Your more youthful face will continue to age, and in 7 to 10 years, you may be ready for a second face-lift.

Multiple Face-Lifts

There is no limit to the number of face-lifts you may have. Multiple face-lifts, however, may cause loss of sideburns or tight face (see "Telltale Signs"). If you are seeking a second or third face-lift, ask how your surgeon preserves sideburns and avoids an unnaturally tight appearance.

Satisfaction

Most women who undergo a face-lift have a reasonable result without complications, and they are typically satisfied.

With many things in life, the greater the degree of improvement, the happier one is for having sought the change. For example, washing a filthy car usually gives greater satisfaction than washing a clean car. Although the final result is the same, a notable change is more gratifying than a subtle one.

Such is the case with face-lifts. The greater your facial sagging, jowls, and neck laxity beforehand, the more dramatic your improvement, and the more satisfied you will be with the procedure. If you are in your 50s, expect a face-lift to subtract 7 to 10 years from your apparent age. If you are 80 years old, a face-lift may subtract 15 years. If you are 35 years old, it may only subtract 5 years.

Concluding Thoughts

Face-lift surgery is the cornerstone of facial rejuvenation. It can tighten lax skin, eliminate jowls, reduce double chins, soften the skin fold of your cheeks, and sharpen the angle between your neck and jawline. Because it does not rejuvenate the eyes, forehead, or facial wrinkles, many women consider other procedures as well—peels, laser resurfacing, eyelid surgery, and forehead lift. So long as you understand what can

MARGARET, *the owner of a small shop, had her first face-lift at 53. She noticed afterward that her sideburns had migrated upward. When she sought her second face-lift, at 61, she did not want to risk further distortion of this feature. She interviewed three plastic surgeons before finding one whose technique would not result in further upward migration of her sideburns. After surgery, she was pleased with her result and glad she still had sideburns.*

EILEEN, *a 73-year-old grandmother, and Debbie, her 43-year-old daughter, both wanted to look younger. They had face-lifts performed on the same day so that they could recover side by side. They had similar facial features, and both were pleased with their results. Although Debbie continued to look much younger than Eileen, Debbie's change was not as dramatic. She was almost envious of her mother's impressive change compared to her own modest change.*

Questions to Ask Your Plastic Surgeon

Will the incision be below or into my hairline?

Will your technique make me look like a different person?

How do you prevent high or absent sideburns?

How do you avoid the wind-tunnel look?

How do you avoid attached earlobes?

be reasonably accomplished by a face-lift, you will likely be satisfied with your results.

Tips and Traps

Because a face-lift will only rejuvenate the lower two-thirds of your face, consider eyelid surgery and forehead lift at the same time, to restore youth and maintain harmony.

Quit smoking two weeks to two months prior to surgery.

Quit taking aspirin and aspirin products at least two weeks before surgery.

Quit taking ibuprofen and related medications three days prior to surgery.

Wait two to three months after a chemical peel or laser resurfacing of your cheeks before you have a face-lift (unless it is a micro peel).

If you are considering a deep face-lift (subperiosteal or cheek lift), anticipate prolonged swelling (three weeks to six months) and an alteration of your basic facial appearance. Understand that the older you are, the more difficult it will be for you to adapt to your new appearance.

Sleep in a recliner or with your head elevated on pillows for the first several days to minimize swelling. Apply ice frequently.

Expect that your face-lift will turn back the clock by about 7 to 10 years. Your face will continue to age, and you may be ready for another lift within a decade.

Know that repeat face-lifts confer a higher risk of leaving you with telltale signs.

3

Raising Your Eyebrows

Forehead Lift

$\mathcal{M}$any of our facial expressions are determined by the appearance of our foreheads and eyebrows. In the operating room, doctors and nurses wear masks that cover their noses and mouths, allowing only their eyes and foreheads to be seen. However, their emotions are hardly concealed. The eyes and forehead alone can reveal if a person is happy, laughing, uncertain, anxious, angry, or contemplative.

DONNA, *a pleasant 69-year-old, was told by others that she looked angry even though she was a cheerful woman who was seldom irritated. One day, her 7-year-old granddaughter said, "Nanny, why are you always so mad at me?" Not surprisingly, she sought plastic surgery within a week. Following a forehead lift, her scowl line softened and her unintended frown faded.*

An aging forehead with low brows and deep creases can make a person appear tired or angry. Changing the eyebrows and forehead can have a dramatic effect. Many plastic surgeons find forehead lift, also called brow lift, to be a more powerful tool in facial rejuvenation than facelift.

The Good News: Things a Forehead Lift Can Improve

A forehead lift will improve brow position, lateral hoods, horizontal forehead wrinkles, and scowl lines (fig. 3-1).

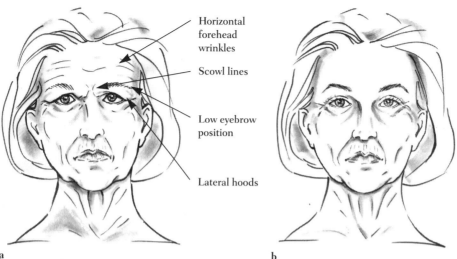

Horizontal
forehead
wrinkles

Scowl lines

Low eyebrow
position

Lateral hoods

a   b

Figure 3-1: *The effects of a forehead lift. (a) Features of an aging face. (b) After a forehead lift the furrows are gone, the horizontal forehead lines are softened, the eyebrows are higher, and the hoods have been minimized. The crow's feet, excess eyelid skin, puffy eyelids, and the rest of the face are unchanged.*

Brow Position

Put your finger on your eyebrow and press inward toward the bone. Feel for the position of the bony rim above your eye. If your eyebrow position is ideal, it will be above the bony rim of your eye socket. If it has descended, it will be below the rim. While looking in the mirror, place your thumb and index finger on your forehead and lift your forehead skin up against the bone. You will see the effect a forehead lift can achieve. Forehead lift will raise your brow to the level of your bony rim or above.

There are two reasons for low brow position: age and genetics. As we age, our skin and soft tissues lose elasticity. This makes them more susceptible to the pull of gravity. Yet, aging is not the only reason the brows may be low. Some women inherit low eyebrows. These women often seek forehead lift in their 20s and 30s.

Lateral Hoods

Lateral hoods are folds of skin between the eyebrow and the eyelid near the outside corner of the eye. They are named for the hooded appearance they give the

Alex, *a 33-year-old police detective, felt she had two strikes against her when it came to meeting new people: her serious job and her serious appearance. This combination made her seem intense and unapproachable. Her serious air stemmed from her low eyebrows—a family curse. Following a forehead lift, her appearance softened, and she felt as though her appearance more closely reflected her lighthearted personality. "It was a good thing the forehead lift helped me," she said laughingly, "because I really didn't want to change careers."*

eyes. Study your face in the mirror. If you have lateral hoods, you will notice improvement in them when you use your finger to lift your forehead.

Lateral hoods are natural by-products of aging and contribute significantly to an aged and tired appearance. Many hope their lateral hoods will be remedied by eyelid surgery, but they will not. Only a forehead lift will improve this problem.

Horizontal Forehead Wrinkles

Looking in the mirror, raise your eyebrows and note the deep creases across your forehead. Relax your eyebrows and watch the creases soften. The creases are a direct result of your repeated efforts to raise your eyebrows. Since your eyebrows descend with age, you use your forehead muscle progressively more, and the problem worsens over time. A forehead lift elevates your brow, allows your forehead muscle to relax, and reduces your horizontal wrinkles. If you have low eyebrows and deep horizontal forehead creases, you probably look tired and may improve your appearance through a forehead lift.

Since 1997, many have sought Botox injections to soften or eliminate horizontal forehead creases, scowl lines, and crow's feet. Botox weakens the muscles responsible for causing wrinkles, thereby allowing them to soften and fade. Horizontal forehead wrinkles are caused by the frontalis muscle, which raises the eyebrows. Thus, injection of this muscle to decrease wrinkles will also disable eyebrow raising.

Because women with severely droopy eyebrows constantly and unconsciously try to raise them, Botox injection will confound their efforts, and their eyebrows may appear droopier. Women with mild to moderate brow droop are not as likely to suffer this consequence because they do not constantly keep their eyebrows raised. (See Chapter 11 for a more thorough discussion of Botox.)

EDITH, *a 66-year-old newspaper editor, was told by her reporters that she always had a disapproving look when she read their articles. Although the articles were not perfect, they did not deserve the scowls their authors thought they evoked. Edith did not intend her harsh facial expressions and sought to remedy her scowls and deep forehead creases. However, she did not want surgery. She tried Botox injections. Although the injections improved her wrinkles, they caused her frontalis muscle to relax, thereby allowing her brows to droop further. She finally had a forehead lift and was satisfied with improvement in her wrinkles and brow position.*

Scowl Lines

While looking in the mirror, try to frown or look angry. You will drive your eyebrows downward and inward toward your nose, creating furrows and vertical wrinkles between your brows. If you have well-developed scowl lines, they can be seen without frowning because the muscles that cause them have been well-conditioned through repetitive use. This is referred to as an unconscious frown because it lends an unintended angry expression. A forehead lift aims to diminish the muscles responsible for scowling, thereby diminishing the vertical wrinkles between the eyebrows and eliminating the angry look.

The Bad News: Things a Forehead Lift Cannot Improve

Look in the mirror again. Close one eye while leaving the other eye open. You will see excess skin on your closed upper eyelid. This skin is usually so redundant that you can probably pinch it between two fingers while still closing your eye. As you lift your forehead up against the bone, you will notice that only some of this excess skin is tightened. Most excess upper eyelid skin will not be affected by a forehead lift. Nor will eyelid puffiness. To remedy these problems, you will need eyelid surgery (Chapter 4).

While looking in the mirror, squint. You will see wrinkles on the outside of your eyes, called crow's feet. Crow's feet will not be improved by forehead lift. Nor will they be improved by eyelid surgery. (See Chapters 11 and 12 for options in treating crow's feet.)

RHONDA, a 40-year-old attorney, disliked the deep furrow between her eyebrows. It seemed to worsen every year she practiced law. She loved the effect Botox had on her furrows but soon tired of repeated injections. She wanted a more permanent fix. A forehead lift both improved her scowl lines and lifted her brows, giving her a softer and more energetic appearance.

The Good News About Forehead Lifts

- *Brow position can be elevated.*
- *Lateral hoods can be reduced.*
- *Horizontal forehead wrinkles can be softened.*
- *Scowl lines between the eyebrows can be improved.*

Other Procedures to Consider

Because the entire face ages at once, and because a forehead lift will rejuvenate only your forehead, you may also seek a face-lift and eyelid surgery. These may be performed at the same time or at a later date.

Forehead lift will improve forehead wrinkles to varying degrees depending on wrinkle severity and the surgical technique. To maximize wrinkle reduction, you may consider Botox injection, laser resurfacing, or chemical peel in addition to forehead lift (Chapters 11 and 12).

How It Works

The goals of a forehead lift are to raise your eyebrows to a higher position, to reduce lateral hoods, and to soften horizontal forehead wrinkles and vertical scowl lines. These goals are accomplished by shifting your forehead skin upward and by affecting the muscles responsible for causing wrinkles and scowl lines.

Your horizontal wrinkles are due to raising your eyebrows via your frontalis muscle. A forehead lift reduces the need to raise your eyebrows (see "Horizontal Forehead Wrinkles"). Some procedures also alter the frontalis muscle directly, thereby weakening it.

Meanwhile, your vertical scowl lines are due to repetitive scowling, via the corrugator and procerus muscles, located above your nose and eyebrows. All forehead lift techniques weaken these scowl muscles, allowing the furrow to soften and the vertical wrinkles to fade.

Forehead Lift Techniques

Lifting the forehead skin and altering the forehead can be accomplished through three different surgical techniques: endoscopic, coronal, and subcutaneous. Each has advantages and disadvantages. You and your plastic surgeon will select the most appropriate one based on which advantages are most important to you and which disadvantages you can most easily accept.

Some surgeons modify one of these three techniques or combine two techniques. Often such approaches (like those described in this chapter) have more than one name.

Endoscopic Lift

Endoscopic forehead lift is the most common technique. It is also the most recently developed one, having been widely used only since 1994.

Endoscopic surgery enables your surgeon to view the procedure with a tiny camera, the size of an eraser head, inserted under your skin. The surgeon makes four to six small incisions hidden behind the hairline (fig. 3-2, solid short lines). Then skin is

---

ARLENE, *a 58-year-old concert violinist, had eyelid surgery and was angry because she felt her upper eyelids were still baggy. She complained to her surgeon about this, but he refused to remove any more skin. Instead, he recommended a forehead lift. Frustrated, Arlene sought a second opinion from me. After examining her, I told her that her first surgeon was correct. She had had an excellent result and would need a forehead lift for further improvement. Having expected me to disagree with her surgeon, she was somewhat surprised and confused. To explain, I asked her to look in a mirror as I pulled her eyebrows up. She immediately recognized that this maneuver solved her problem of apparent excess upper eyelid skin. She realized her problem was one of droopy eyebrows, not excess eyelid skin. She further realized that if she had convinced her first surgeon to remove more skin, that a subsequent forehead lift would have prevented her from closing her eyes. A forehead lift solved her problem of apparent excess eyelid skin without compromising the function of her eyelids.*

The Bad News About Forehead Lifts

- *Baggy eyelids will not be improved.*
- *Puffy eyes will not be improved.*
- *Crow's feet will not be improved.*

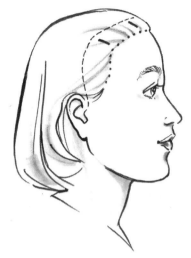 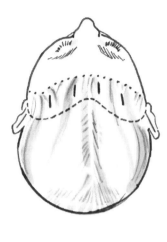

FIGURE 3-2: *Forehead lift incisions. The* endoscopic *forehead lift involves four to six small incisions, hidden behind the hairline (short solid lines). The* coronal *forehead lift involves a single long incision from one ear to the other, behind the hairline (dashed line). The* subcutaneous *forehead lift involves a single long incision on top of the forehead, at the hairline (dotted line).*

shifted backward on the head. To ensure temporary support for the skin until it has healed in its new location, some surgeons place drill holes or small screws into the skull. Finally they place sutures around the screws or through the holes to anchor the skin. (If metal screws are used, they will be removed in the office two weeks later. If absorbable screws are used, they will dissolve within a few months.)

Endoscopic lift has several distinct advantages. Large incisions are avoided. Temporary numbness on the top of the scalp (which always occurs following coronal lift) is not usually a problem.

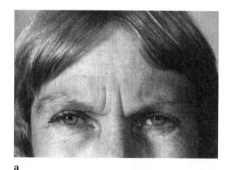 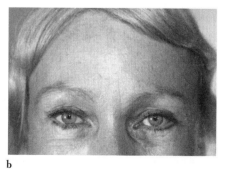

a   b

(a) Before endoscopic forehead lift. (b) After endoscopic forehead lift. Note the softer overall appearance and the absence of the unintended scowl.

BETTY, *a 45-year-old florist, had moderate aging and average forehead height. She did not want the numbness or the long scar associated with a coronal forehead lift. Because she wore her hair off her face, she did not want the hairline scar associated with a subcutaneous lift. She chose to have an endoscopic forehead lift and was pleased with her decision.*

Typically, you can expect 50 to 75 percent improvement in each forehead wrinkle after an endoscopic lift. Most will still be present, but all will be improved. If you seek laser or chemical peel of your forehead for further improvement of wrinkles, these can be safely performed on the same day.

The endoscopic forehead lift also has disadvantages. It will raise your hairline by about one-half inch, which may be a problem for those with high foreheads before surgery. Although screw and drill hole placement is safe, some women are uncomfortable with this idea. Also, because the frontalis muscle is not altered, women who use their forehead expressively may find that horizontal lines are barely improved and quick to return. And those with overwhelming descent of the brow or deep creases will likely be disappointed with an endoscopic lift because they will find it to be less effective and shorter lasting than the other options.

Generally, women with minimal to moderate forehead aging and an average hairline height prefer this technique to the other two (see Table 3-1).

If you are having eyelid surgery at the same time as your forehead lift, your surgeon may use your upper eyelid incisions to perform more work on your scowl muscles. If so, temporary lid droop may occur as well as more swelling and bruising. Recovery time will be about two weeks longer. Many surgeons feel they are able to get the same improvement in vertical scowl lines using the endoscopic incisions alone. Ask about your surgeon's plans.

Coronal Lift

In a coronal forehead lift, the incision extends across the top of the head from ear to ear (fig. 3-2, dashed line). All muscles of the forehead are surgically

Endoscopic Lift

ADVANTAGES	DISADVANTAGES
1. Small incisions.	1. Poor results in advanced aging.
2. Good result for minimal to moderate forehead aging.	2. Raises the hairline.
3. Chemical peel, laser, or dermabrasion can be safely performed on the same day.	3. Drill holes or screws may be used to temporarily support the brow in its new position.

Table 3-1 *Comparison of Techniques*

	Endoscopic	Cornal	Subcutaneous
Site of incision?	Multiple small incisions behind hairline	Incision from ear to ear across top of head	Incision across top of forehead
Scalp numbness?	Rarely	Yes, lasts about 6 months	Rarely
Raises hairline?	Yes	Yes	No
Requires attachment to to skull?	Sometimes	No	No
Risk of recurrent forehead droop?	Some	Rare	Rare
Effect on horizontal wrinkles?	Mild to moderate	Dramatic	Dramatic
Effect on vertical scowl lines?	Moderate	Moderate	Moderate
Safe to have forehead laser or peel at same time?	Yes	Yes	No
Who should not have this operation?	Those with severe brow droop, deep horizontal creases, or a high hairline	Those with a high hairline	Those who wear their hair off their face, smokers, and those seeking forehead peel/laser at the same time.
Ideal candidate for this procedure?	Those with mild to moderate aging of their forehead	Those with severe aging: major eyebrow droop and deep horizontal wrinkles	Those with a high forehead who wear their hair forward
Popularity	Most common	Second most common	Third most common

weakened. Then the surgeon lifts the forehead to its desired position. At that point, the scalp in front of the incision overlaps the scalp behind it. After removing the overlapping scalp the surgeon sews the remaining scalp together.

MARY, *a 79-year-old widow with advanced forehead aging, desired a forehead lift, eyelid surgery, and a facelift. Because of her advanced wrinkles, deep furrows, and very low brows, she had a coronal lift for the maximal effect. An endoscopic lift would not give her enough improvement, and she did not want a subcutaneous lift because she wore her hair back.*

ANN, *a 62-year-old nonsmoker with heavy brows and deep wrinkles, wore bangs over her face and had a high forehead. She chose the subcutaneous lift for a few reasons. An endoscopic lift would not have provided as much improvement, and a coronal lift would have shifted her hairline back further. Because she wore her hair forward, her hairline scar was hidden.*

Coronal lifts offer several advantages. All muscles that contribute to wrinkles and scowling can be altered, including the frontalis muscle, which is responsible for deep horizontal creases. Screws are not necessary, and the lift may last longer than with endoscopic technique. Typically the well-hidden scar is not detectable. This technique offers an excellent aesthetic result, particularly in women with severe descent of the brows and deep forehead creases.

Expect that each wrinkle will improve by 90 percent. Because of the dramatic results, few need chemical peel or laser resurfacing of their foreheads. (However, if you and your surgeon thought these additional treatments were appropriate, any of them could be safely performed.)

Coronal lifts impose several disadvantages. Numbness and itching behind the scar on top of the head can last for six months. The scar is long, which is considered a disadvantage by some. As with the endoscopic lift, your hairline will be raised following surgery, which can be a problem if you have a high forehead.

Generally, women with advanced forehead droop and an average hairline height prefer this procedure to the other two techniques.

Subcutaneous ("Skin-Only") Lift

The incision for a subcutaneous forehead lift is just below the hairline (fig. 3-2, dotted line).

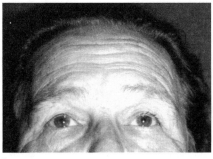 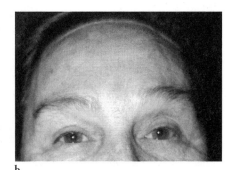

a   b

(a) Before subcutaneous forehead lift. (b) After subcutaneous forehead lift. Note the scar at the top of the forehead.

Subcutaneous lifts can offer several real advantages. Because the incision is in front of the hairline, the hairline is not shifted upward when skin is removed. In contrast to coronal lift, the sensory nerves to the top of the head are not divided, and problems with numbness and itching are uncommon. Improvement in horizontal creases is dramatic, just as in a coronal lift.

The main disadvantage is a visible scar along the hairline, a concern for women who wear their hair back. The scar may heal imperceptibly, but this can neither be predicted nor guaranteed. Laser procedures and chemical peels cannot be safely performed at the same time as the subcutaneous lift due to concern over circulation to the skin. Skin circulation is compromised more with subcutaneous lift than with endoscopic or coronal lift because of technical details pertaining to the procedure. Therefore, smokers will have more healing problems with this technique than other techniques.

Women who have a high forehead and are willing to accept a scar along the hairline may prefer this technique to the other two.

What to Expect

Forehead lifts are commonly performed under sedation anesthesia, and you will be allowed to go home the same day, provided someone else drives. Discomfort is mild and will be controlled with acetaminophen (Tylenol) or a mild prescription pain medication. You will be presentable in public with the help of makeup within two weeks. Your final result will be evident within four weeks.

To help you to plan for and recover from your procedure reread Steps 7 and 10 of Chapter 1.

Complications

When your operation is performed by a qualified plastic surgeon, both your procedure and recovery will likely be uneventful. Even in ideal circumstances, how-

---

Vital Statistics

Anesthesia: Sedation or general.

Location of operation: Office or hospital.

Length of surgery: 30–90 minutes.

Length of stay: Outpatient (home same day).

Discomfort: Mild; anticipate 0–4 days of prescription pain medication. Many take only Tylenol.

Swelling and bruising: Improve in 10–14 days. You can reduce swelling through constant head elevation and frequent application of ice. You may develop black eyes temporarily.

Bandages: Removed in 1–3 days.

Stitches: Removed in 7–10 days. If your surgeon placed metal screws in your skull (for endoscopic lift), they will be removed in 2–3 weeks.

Contact lenses: May be worn in 1 week.

Makeup: May be worn in 3–5 days.

Presentable in public: 7–14 days, with the help of makeup.

Work: You may feel capable of returning within 3 days, but your appearance will be the limiting factor.

Exercise: May be resumed in 2 weeks.

Final result: Seen in 2–4 weeks.

ever, complications may occur. In addition to the specific complications mentioned here, refer to Chapter 1 for an explanation of general complications that may occur with any procedure.

Forehead Paralysis

Paralysis of one side of the forehead occurs in fewer than 1 percent of patients and is due to nerve damage. It is usually temporary and full motion usually returns within three months.

If forehead motion fails to return within six months, it is likely permanent. Cases of permanent paralysis are obvious and disfiguring. During facial expression, only the normal side moves, and at rest only the normal side has wrinkles.

Surgical restoration of a paralyzed forehead will not be possible for the foreseeable future. Because symmetric paralysis is less obvious than one-sided paralysis, treatment involves damaging the nerve on the normal side of the forehead. Intentional paralysis can be created through Botox injections or by surgically cutting the nerve.

Brow Asymmetry

After forehead lift, your new brow position may appear higher on one side than the other. In most cases, the asymmetry was present before surgery. Therefore, it is important for you and your surgeon to recognize any asymmetry and discuss it prior to surgery. Asymmetry can be managed in two ways. The first option is for your surgeon to lift both brows to the same level. This may seem ideal, but if you have become accustomed to looking at your asymmetric brows for decades, as most have, then you may have difficulty adjusting to your new symmetric look. As noted in Chapter 1, everyone is asymmetric. Maintaining your asymmetry, therefore, is a second, reasonable option.

Permanent Loss of Hair

Following coronal or endoscopic lifts, small bald spots may occur along the scar line. If your hair fails to grow back, you may either comb your hair over the bald spot, have hair transplanted to fill the bald spot, or ask your plastic surgeon to surgically remove the bald spot. If your surgeon removes the bald spot, the surrounding hair-bearing skin will be sutured together, leaving a small scar that will be hidden in your hair.

When Can I Stop Worrying About Complications?

Most complications occur within a predictable time following surgery. If you do not develop them within the time periods noted, you can fairly conclude that you are probably free of these complications:

Time Since Surgery	Possible Complication
1 day	*Paralysis*
1 day	*Numbness*
3 months	*Brow asymmetry*
3 months	*Permanent hair loss*
6 months	*Early relapse*

Numbness

As previously mentioned, temporary numbness on the top of the head is expected following a coronal lift. Numbness of the entire forehead, however, can occur with any technique when there has been damage to the sensory nerves. These nerves emerge through the forehead bone directly above the eye and run through the scowl muscles. Because the scowl muscles are removed or modified during surgery, these nerves are at risk for being stretched, cut, or burned.

Numbness of the forehead can occur temporarily or permanently if the sensory nerve is injured. In cases of temporary numbness, sensation usually returns within two weeks but may not return for three months. If permanent numbness occurs, sensation cannot be restored. Risk of permanent numbness is less than 1 percent. If this rare complication occurs, you will likely become accustomed to it within a year.

Early Relapse

Early relapse means that your brow drops again within a few months. This may occur after endoscopic lift if your forehead was inadequately suspended at the time of surgery. Because screws and drill holes are now commonly employed, this problem has become rare. Early relapse does not usually occur after coronal or subcutaneous forehead lift.

Telltale Signs

Unnatural Facial Expression

If your eyebrows are not raised in harmony to a natural level, unnatural facial expressions can result. The brows may be raised to an artificially high position, leaving you with a surprised look (fig. 3-3). If the inner half of your eyebrow is raised more than the outer half, a sad appearance may occur (fig. 3-4a). If the outer half is raised more than the inner half, a strange look may result (fig. 3-4b). The brows may spread apart, creating an unnaturally wide gap between them. Some of these problems can be corrected through further surgery, others cannot. The best way to prevent these problems is through selection of a qualified plastic surgeon.

Visible Scar

When subcutaneous lift is performed, the scar may be visible if you wear your hair pulled back off your face. Avoid this technique if you are unwilling to wear bangs.

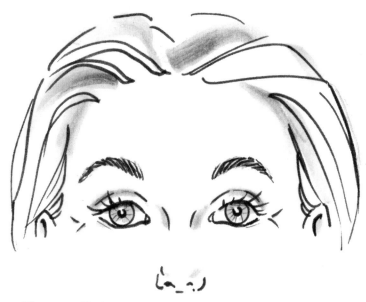

FIGURE 3-3: *The surprised look is a telltale sign that results after the eyebrows have been excessively raised. This problem is difficult to correct.*

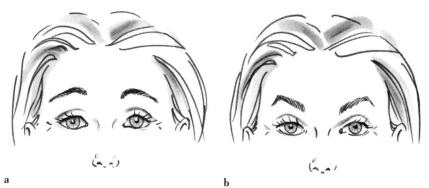

a   b

FIGURE 3-4: *(a) Eyebrows with excessively raised inner portion result in a telltale sad appearance.
(b) Eyebrows with excessively raised outer portion result in a strange telltale appearance.*

High Hairline (High Forehead)

An unnaturally high hairline can occur in those who have high hairlines before a forehead lift. If a technique other than the subcutaneous one is used, your hairline will be shifted further upward, creating an unnatural appearance (fig. 3-5). This can be avoided by choosing a subcutaneous lift if you have a high hairline.

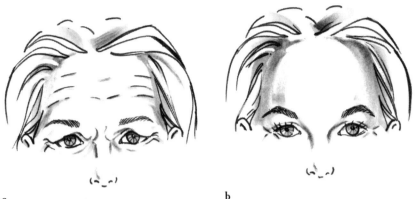

a   b

FIGURE 3-5: *(a) A high hairline before forehead lift. (b) Following either endoscopic or coronal lift, an already high hairline can appear unnaturally high.*

Muscle Bulges

Small soft bulges may occur above your nose between your eyebrows following surgery. These result from incomplete removal of the scowling muscles and can be corrected through revision brow surgery or Botox injections.

Cost

In the United States, the range of total fees for a forehead lift extends from $3,000 to $5,000. The average cost is:

Surgeon's fee	$2,600
Anesthesiologist's fee	$ 600
Operating room (facility) fee	$ 800
Total	$4,000

See "Fees" in Chapter 1 for various factors that might affect your own actual cost.

Duration of Results

The duration of a forehead lift depends on the technique used. Coronal or subcutaneous lifts are lasting and rarely need to be repeated.

Because endoscopic lift is a newer technique, the duration of results are not yet known. With time and gravity, your forehead may re-descend and require another forehead lift. This will occur sooner in those with advanced aging of the forehead and is one reason for those with severely low brows and deep creases to opt for a different technique. Long-term results cannot be determined until a technique has been used for several decades.

Young Women with Low Brows

A few women inherit low eyebrows. These women may undergo successful forehead lift in young adulthood. As they age, they will gradually develop forehead wrinkles and droopy brows. They may then seek a second forehead lift later in life regardless of the technique used for the first lift.

Satisfaction

As with many plastic surgery procedures, satisfaction following a forehead lift is tied to the degree of improvement. Those with advanced droop of their brows and deep creases are likely to see greater change than those with more subtle signs of aging. Regardless of the starting point, all will see some improvement in brow position, horizontal forehead wrinkles, and scowl lines. Because forehead lift improves lateral hoods, it can also enhance the appearance of the upper eyelids. However, some women are disappointed due to inflated expectations, complications, telltale signs, or recurrence of forehead droop. Most are reasonably satisfied with their results, provided their expectations were realistic.

Questions to Ask Your Plastic Surgeon

Do I need eyelid surgery too?

Which technique do you recommend in my case?

If endoscopic surgery is planned, how will you secure my new brow position?

Can you correct my brow asymmetry?

Where will the incisions be?

Concluding Thoughts

An aging upper face can cause you to unintentionally appear tired or angry. Forehead lift involves raising your brows and altering the underlying muscles to soften your appearance. Depending on the severity of your problem, the height of your forehead, and your hairstyle, one of several techniques may be chosen and tailored to your needs.

Among all facial rejuvenation procedures, forehead lift can have the most dramatic effect on overall appearance.

Tips and Traps

Quit taking aspirin and ibuprofen for two weeks and three days, respectively, prior to surgery. Discuss all of your nonprescription medications with your doctor.

If you have mild to moderate brow droop and horizontal wrinkles, an endoscopic lift may be most appropriate.

If you have advanced brow droop with deep wrinkles, a coronal forehead lift may be most appropriate.

If you have a high forehead, regardless of the degree of brow droop and wrinkles, and if you wear your hair forward, a subcutaneous forehead lift may be most appropriate.

Anticipate that your forehead will look higher after an endoscopic or coronal lift than it did before surgery.

A forehead lift will not improve your baggy eyelids or crow's feet.

Sleep in a recliner or with your head elevated on pillows for the first several days after surgery to minimize swelling. Apply ice compresses frequently!

4

Rejuvenating Your Eyes

Eyelid Surgery

Our eyes are focal points of our faces because they are central to communication. When we speak, we look each other in the eye. When we wish to better understand one another, when we ask questions, and when we search for answers, we look into the eyes of the other person. Much emphasis is therefore placed on the appearance of the eyes.

Eyelid surgery, or *blepharoplasty,* is the third most commonly performed cosmetic procedures in the United States (after liposuction and breast augmentation). Before exploring the changes that eyelid surgery can accomplish, it is helpful to understand the aesthetic goal of eyelid surgery.

JOYCE, *a 63-year-old widow, was alone for several years before meeting and falling in love with a man eight years her junior. Self-conscious about their age difference, she wanted to close the apparent gap. She underwent eyelid surgery, which restored a more energetic and youthful appearance. Thereafter, she felt more at ease when they were together in public.*

The Ideal Eyelid

With an aesthetically ideal eyelid (fig. 4-1), the upper lid rests just below the top of the iris, which is the colored ring around the pupil. The lower lid rests just above the lower border of the iris. Hence, the white of the eye should be seen neither above nor below the iris. If it is, the eye will appear as though it is bulging out of the socket. The ideal eyelid has no excess skin, no puffiness, and strong tone (see "Self-Evaluation for Lower Lid Laxity" later in this chapter).

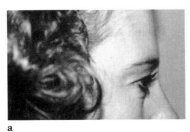
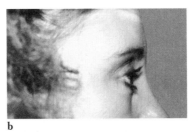

a   **b**

(a) Before upper and lower eyelid surgery. (b) After upper and lower eyelid surgery.

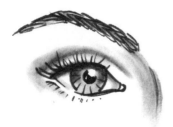
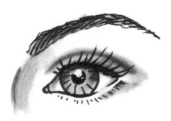

FIGURE 4-1: *Aesthetically ideal eyes. Note the position of the eyelids as they relate to the iris. (The iris is the colored ring around the pupil.)*

The Good News: Things Eyelid Surgery Will Improve

Most cosmetic eyelid surgery is performed to correct bagginess and puffiness of the eyelids, and sometimes lid position is altered as well. Changes in ethnicity are less common. All of these are described below. (See fig. 4-2.)

Excess Skin of the Eyelids (Baggy Eyelids)

Excess skin of the eyelids creates a heavy and tired appearance. Look in the mirror and close one eye while leaving the other eye open. Using your thumb and index finger, pinch the extra skin of your closed upper eyelid. The amount of skin that you can easily pinch between your thumb and finger with your eye closed is the amount of skin that can be removed from the upper eyelids during eyelid surgery. Excess skin of the lower eyelid, if it exists, can be seen without special maneuvers.

Protruding Fat of the Eyelids (Puffy Eyelids)

It is normal to have fat surrounding your eyeball. But, over time, this fat may protrude into the eyelids, creating puffiness. Surprisingly, this is not related to weight gain, and weight loss cannot be expected to improve puffiness. It is simply related to genetics and aging. Removing fat through eyelid surgery will reduce puffiness.

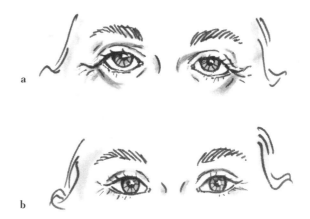

FIGURE 4-2: *The effects of eyelid surgery. (a) Eyelid bagginess, puffiness, upper lid droopiness, and lower lid laxity. (b) Eyelid surgery will correct these problems, but will not affect crow's feet, furrows, brow position, or lateral hoods.*

Some young women have puffy eyelids and may seek surgery in young adulthood. They invariably have mothers or sisters with the same problem. They have an inherited predisposition for eyelid fat to protrude early in life. Because young women usually have no excess skin, they are good candidates for fat removal alone.

Look in the mirror and close one eye. While gently pressing on your eye through the closed upper lid, watch the skin above and below that eye. If the skin above and below your closed eye bulges while you are pressing, then you probably have protruding fat as a cause of your puffy eyelids and would benefit from removal of fat during eyelid surgery.

Droopy Upper Eyelids

Look in the mirror. Pay careful attention to the lower edge of your upper eyelid. It should fall just below the top of your iris, which is the colored part of your eye. You should be able to see most of the iris above the pupil, but not the very top of it (fig. 4-1). If the lower edge of your upper eyelid blocks more than the very top of your iris, then your upper eyelid is droopy (fig. 4-3). Plastic surgeons call this condition *eyelid ptosis*. The "p" is silent.

In some cases, droopiness is so severe that the edge of the upper eyelid encroaches upon the pupil and interferes with vision. Those with droopiness of the upper

MELISSA, *a 32-year-old stay-at-home mom, was frustrated that her eyes appeared puffy. Her friends of similar age did not have this problem. Following eyelid surgery during which only fat was removed, her puffiness was gone. Not surprisingly, her sister had the same eyelid problem and requested the same procedure six months later.*

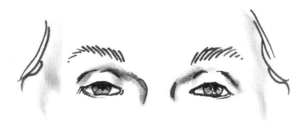

FIGURE 4-3: *Droopy upper eyelids. The upper eyelid covers some of the pupil and more of the iris than normal.*

eyelid are often told that they look tired or that their eyes appear small. The most common cause of eyelid droop is weakness or detachment of the muscle responsible for holding the eyelid open. This typically occurs with aging but can also be an inherited trait. Therefore, young women may have this problem.

Lax (Loose) Lower Eyelids

Lax lower eyelids means they are loose. If laxity is mild, it may cause dry eye symptoms but the lids will look normal. If laxity is severe, dry eye symptoms may be debilitating, and the lids may look droopy. Severely lax lower lids droop below the iris, allowing the white of the eye to be seen between the pupil and the lid.

Looking in the mirror, pay careful attention to the position of the upper edge of your lower eyelid. It should rest just above the lower border of your iris so that you can see no white below your iris. If you can see the white of your eye, also called the sclera, below the iris, your lower lid laxity is severe (fig. 4-4). If your lower lid position appears normal, you may still have mild laxity.

Any degree of laxity must be recognized prior to surgery so that it can be repaired. Untreated laxity will worsen as a result of eyelid surgery.

You can determine yourself whether your lower eyelids are loose (see "Self-Evaluation for Lower Eyelid Laxity").

To correct laxity, a simple procedure called *canthopexy* may be performed with your eyelid surgery. Canthopexy tightens your lower eyelids—preventing droopiness and averting dry eye symptoms. Your sur-

VICTORIA, *a delightful 72-year-old woman, made an appointment for a consultation stating that her eyes were too small. The morning of her consultation, I reviewed the list of patients and their concerns. I remember seeing her concern and thinking that I had no idea how to make eyeballs bigger—nor did I know anyone who did. When she came in, I was relieved to discover that she did not want her eyeballs enlarged. She just wanted the opening between her eyelids widened. When I told her what I had at first thought she wanted, we both laughed. She had significant droop of her upper eyelids with only a narrow slit through which to see the world. She underwent eyelid surgery and ptosis repair with improvement in her appearance. I now see her about once a year, and each time she jokingly reminds me to leave her eyeballs alone.*

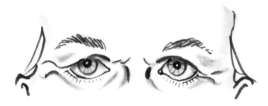

FIGURE 4-4: *Droopy lower eyelids. Severe lower lid laxity appears as droopy lower eyelids. The white of the eye can be seen below the iris.*

geon should assess eyelid position and tone to determine your need for this procedure. If canthopexy is recommended, you should agree to it. (Some plastic surgeons may charge extra for this.)

Asian Eyelids

Caucasians have an upper eyelid crease about one-third of an inch above their eyelashes. Asians do not have this crease, because the fibers that form this skin crease in Caucasians are not present. Some Asians seek a Caucasian appearing eyelid. Their eyelids can be modified to appear Caucasian by surgically creating an attachment between the muscle and the upper eyelid skin about one-third of an inch above the eyelashes (fig. 4-5). This can be done in conjunction with eyelid surgery or as an independent procedure.

Alternatively, it is possible to convert a Caucasian eyelid into an Asian eyelid by surgically disrupting the attachments between the muscle and the eyelid skin.

Self-Evaluation for Lower Eyelid Laxity

1. *Look in the mirror at the inner and outer corners of your eye. The outer corner should be slightly higher than the inner corner. If they are at the same level, you may have mild laxity. If the outer corner is lower than the inner corner, you may have moderate or severe laxity.*

2. *Distraction test: Place your index finger on your lower eyelid near the lash line and press the lid downward against your facial bone. If you can pull it one-half inch away from your eyeball, you have lower lid laxity.*

3. *Snap-back test: Pinch your lower eyelid between your thumb and forefinger and pull it away from your eyeball. When you release the eyelid, it should snap back to the eyeball briskly and immediately. If not, you have laxity.*

4. *If you can see white below your iris, then you have severe lower lid laxity.*

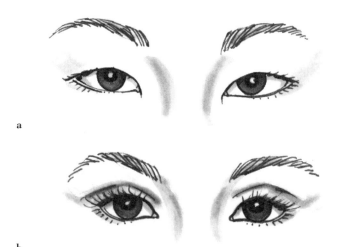

a

b

FIGURE 4-5: *Asian eyelids. (a) Eyelids before surgery. (b) Eyelids after surgery. Note that eyelid surgery does not necessarily alter ethnic traits, unless so desired by the patient.*

The Bad News: Things Eyelid Surgery May Not Improve

Dark Circles

Dark circles under your eyes may be caused by shadows or skin discoloration. If your dark circles are due to shadows, eyelid surgery may help. If they are due to discoloration, eyelid surgery alone will not help.

Shadows, when present, are due to puffy lower eyelids, which in turn are due to fat bulges. Puffy eyelids protrude and caste a shadow below them. To determine if your dark circles are due to discoloration or shadows, study your eyelids in the mirror. Using your index and long fingers, stretch the skin of your lower eyelid. If the dark circles disappear, then they were due to the shadow caste by fat bulges of your lower eyelids and may improve following lower eyelid surgery. If the dark circles remain, they are due to skin discoloration and will not improve following eyelid surgery. Chemical peels or laser resurfacing can sometimes improve discoloration (see Chapter 12).

Some plastic surgeons warn that regardless of the cause of your dark circles, they may actually worsen following surgery. Shadows may worsen if the light reflection under your eyes changes unfavorably due to

CARLA, *a 24-year-old sportswear model, was tall and beautiful but very self-conscious of her lack of upper eyelid creases. She was of Chinese descent and worried that her eyelids prevented her from securing some modeling jobs. She desperately wanted her eyelids modified, but realized that a change in her ethnic appearance might offend her parents. After winning reluctant approval from her parents, she had surgery. She was satisfied with the change in her appearance, and even happier that she had discussed her plans with her family in advance.*

your facial characteristics. Discoloration may worsen due to the trauma of surgery.

Crow's Feet

Crow's feet will not be improved through eyelid surgery. These are wrinkles that can be treated with laser surgery, chemical peels, or Botox. See Chapters 11 and 12 for details.

Droopy Eyebrows and Scowl Lines

Your eyebrows and the furrow between them will not be affected by eyelid surgery. These require a forehead lift.

Lateral Hoods

Lateral hoods are folds of skin between the eyebrow and the eyelid near the outside corner of the eye. They are named for the hooded appearance they give the eyes. Study your eyes in the mirror. If you have lateral hoods, they may initially appear as though they are due to excess eyelid skin, but they are not. They are due to droopy forehead skin. To prove this to yourself, place your fingers above your eyebrows and lift them up as you look in the mirror (fig. 4-6). As you lift, note the improvement in your lateral hoods. Lateral hoods will not be improved through eyelid surgery. For this, a forehead lift is required.

The Good News About Eyelid Surgery

- *Remove excess skin of the upper and lower eyelids*
- *Improve puffiness of the eyelids due to fat*
- *Improve droopy upper eyelids*
- *Improve lax lower eyelids*
- *Alter ethnic traits of the eyelids*

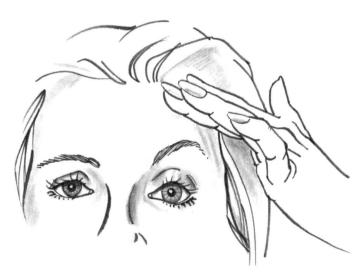

FIGURE 4-6: *The effect of a droopy forehead on baggy eyes. This woman is raising her left eyebrow to demonstrate that a significant portion of her apparent excess eyelid skin is actually due to a droopy forehead.*

As you lift your forehead skin, you will continue to note some excess eyelid skin, although it will appear less abundant than it did when you were not supporting your forehead. The excess skin you see is from your eyelid and will be improved through eyelid surgery.

This exercise is worth repeating because it demonstrates that the excess upper eyelid skin that you perceive is not all truly excess. Typically, only half is due to excess eyelid skin and half is due to droopy eyebrows. In short, if you have both droopy forehead and excess eyelid skin, eyelid surgery alone will likely disappoint you.

Cosmetic Eye Problems Caused by Thyroid Disease

Graves' disease is a thyroid condition that causes the eyes to bulge outward and the eyelids to appear puffy. Some who have Graves' disease but are unaware of its effects mistakenly think that eyelid surgery will improve their appearance. The most appropriate treatment is medical management of the underlying thyroid condition, which may restore a normal appearance to the eyes. If medical management alone fails, then the best surgical procedure may be to enlarge the eye socket. Be leery of a plastic surgeon who proposes eyelid surgery as a treatment for Graves' disease.

The Operation

Eyelid surgery is highly individualized. Some women seek surgery of the upper lids, some seek surgery of the lower lids, and some seek both. Some need skin removal, some need fat removal, and some need both. Some need their lower lids tightened, some need their upper lids raised, and some need both. These determinations are easily made by your plastic surgeon with the maneuvers described earlier. Your operation should be tailored to your needs.

Upper Eyelid Surgery

Upper eyelid surgery is performed through an incision that is designed to remove excess skin. The resultant

---

CATHERINE, *a 62-year-old bridge club champion, requested eyelid surgery. Because of her low brows, eyelid surgery alone would leave her with lateral hoods and apparent excess upper eyelid skin. I also advised her to have a forehead lift for the most improvement. She declined, saying that she would have the forehead lift later . . . if needed. Following eyelid surgery, she complained that she still had excess skin over her upper eyelids. In front of a mirror, I manually lifted her eyebrows. She immediately saw improvement and exclaimed, "That's what I want! Why didn't you do a forehead lift in the first place?"*

Potential Components of Eyelid Surgery

- *Upper eyelid skin removal (for baggy upper eyelids)*

- *Upper eyelid fat removal (for puffy upper eyelids)*

- *Upper eyelid lift (for droopy upper eyelids)*

- *Upper eyelid ethnic modification*

- *Lower eyelid skin removal (for baggy lower eyelids)*

- *Lower eyelid fat removal (for puffy lower eyelids)*

- *Lower eyelid tightening (for lax lower eyelids)*

scar falls along the natural crease of your upper eyelid and will be nearly invisible once it heals (fig. 4-7). Through this incision, upper eyelid fat can be removed, if necessary. Other procedures such as correction of droopy upper eyelids or modification of Asian upper eyelids can be performed through the same incision at the same time.

Correction of upper eyelid droop demands precision, because even a millimeter discrepancy between sides will be obvious. Many plastic surgeons consider this portion of eyelid surgery to be the most challenging.

Lower Eyelid Surgery

Lower eyelid surgery can be performed through one of two incisions. The traditional incision is just below your lower eyelashes and extends out along one of your crow's feet (fig. 4-7). Through this incision, excess skin and fat can be removed if necessary. Lower eyelid tone can be improved at this time through canthopexy, which is performed on the outer corners of the eyes and usually leaves no scars.

The traditional incision heals well and becomes nearly imperceptible within 2 to 4 weeks. When this incision is used, it is unsafe to perform laser or chemical peels at the same time.

The other option is for those who have excess fat of the lower eyelids but no excess skin, such as young women with puffy lower eyelids. The surgeon makes an incision on the inside of the lower eyelid called a transconjunctival incision (fig. 4-8). Through this incision, fat but not skin can be removed from the lower eyelid. This incision is not visible, even immediately

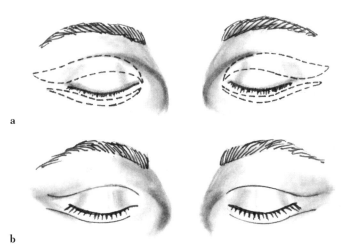

a

b

FIGURE 4-7: *Incisions and scars.(a) The standard incisions for both upper and lower eyelid surgeries (dashed lines). (b) The resultant scar positions (solid lines). Due to the position of the scars and the nature of skin in this area, these scars are usually not visible.*

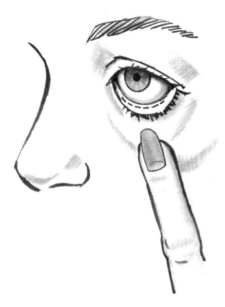

FIGURE 4-8: *Incision on the inside of the lower eyelid. This incision (dashed line) may be used when fat alone is to be removed.*

following surgery. Stitches are unnecessary. When this incision is used, lower eyelid chemical peels and laser resurfacing can be performed safely at the same time.

Laser Eyelid Surgery

Laser eyelid surgery costs several hundred dollars more and yields the same final results as standard surgery. Most plastic surgeons agree that the added expense is not justified.

What to Expect

Eyelid surgery is most commonly performed under sedation anesthesia, and you will be allowed to go home the same day, provided someone else does the driving. Discomfort is mild and will be controlled with Tylenol or mild prescription pain medication. You will be presentable in public with the help of makeup within two weeks. Your final result will be evident within about a month.

To help you to plan for and recover from your procedure, reread Steps 7 and 10 of Chapter 1.

Complications

When your operation is performed by a qualified plastic surgeon, both your procedure and recovery will likely be uneventful. Even in ideal circumstances, however, complications may occur. In addition to the specific complications mentioned here, refer to Chapter 1 for an explanation of general complications that may occur with any procedure.

Blindness

Blindness occurs in less than one in 10,000 who undergo eyelid surgery and is almost always related to bleeding following removal of eyelid fat. Bleeding behind an eyeball pushes it outward and exerts pressure on the retina, causing blindness in that eye. This is rare, but almost always permanent.

Vital Statistics

Anesthesia: General, sedation, or local.

Location of operation: Office or hospital.

Length of surgery: 30–90 minutes.

Length of stay: Outpatient (home same day).

Discomfort: Mild. Anticipate 0–3 days of prescription pain medication or Tylenol. Many require no pain medication.

Swelling and bruising: Improve within 3–14 days depending on the extent of surgery. Following skin removal only, expect 3–5 days. Following skin and fat removal with canthopexy, expect 7–14 days. You can reduce swelling through constant head elevation and frequent application of ice.

Bandages: None. You will be instructed to place ice compresses on your eyes for 1–3 days.

Stitches: Will be removed in 2–4 days. If surgery of the lower lids is performed through the inside of the lids, stitch removal is unnecessary.

Excess tear drops: Expect that your eyes will temporarily be prone to excess tearing, especially when you are outside on a windy day. This typically improves within several weeks.

Contact lenses: May be worn in 7–14 days. Glasses may be worn immediately.

Eye makeup: May be worn in 7–10 days.

Presentable in public: 3–14 days with the help of makeup, depending on the extent of surgery.

Work: You may feel capable of returning within 1–3 days, but your appearance will be the limiting factor.

Exercise: May be resumed in 2 weeks.

Sun protection: 6 months SPF 15 or higher.

Final result: Seen in 2–6 weeks.

Visual Disturbance

Double vision or blurred vision can occur due to damaged eye muscles. It occurs in less than 1 percent of women, is most often temporary, and improves within a few days or weeks. Permanent visual disturbance is rare and may require corrective eye surgery.

Dry Eye Syndrome

Dry eye syndrome is a condition in which the eyes feel dry, gritty, and as though there is sand in them. The eyes are actually watery, and vision is blurred. Although many report these symptoms shortly following eyelid surgery, the eyes should return to normal within a few days or weeks.

Persistent dry eye syndrome can result from lower eyelid surgery; upper eyelid surgery rarely causes it. Symptoms may last for months or years. A number of possible causes exist. Not all are predictable or preventable.

Dry eye syndrome may often be prevented by limiting the amount of skin and fat removed from the lower lids and by tightening the lower lids through a canthopexy procedure.

Treatment for dry eye syndrome depends on the cause. If due to lower lid laxity, it may be improved through canthopexy. If due to removal of too much eyelid skin, it may be improved through skin grafting to the lower lid. If due

When Can I Stop Worrying About Complications?

Most complications occur within a predictable time following surgery. If you do not develop them within the time periods noted, you can fairly conclude that you are probably free of these complications.

TIME SINCE SURGERY	POSSIBLE COMPLICATION
1 day	*Blindness*
1 day	*Blurred or double vision*
1 day	*Dry eye syndrome*
1 day	*Inability to close eyes*
1 day	*Corneal abrasion*
3 months	*Skin cysts*
3 months	*Abnormal lid position*

Causes for Dry Eye Syndrome After Eyelid Surgery

1. Lax lower lid before surgery. *If canthopexy was not performed, your lower lid may be pulled down with resultant dry eye syndrome.*
2. Dry eye tendencies before surgery. *For example, those who are unable to wear contact lenses because their eyes lack adequate moisture are at higher risk for dry eye syndrome.*
3. Preoperative features of flat cheeks and prominent eyes. *For uncertain reasons, this particular anatomy may predispose to dry eye syndrome.*
4. Removal of too much lower eyelid skin during surgery. *Excess skin removal will result in the lower eyelid being pulled downward.*
5. Bad luck. *Dry eye syndrome may occur for no known reason.*

to another cause, your surgeon may have nothing to offer, but your symptoms may improve over time.

Inability to Close Your Eyes

If you are unable to close your eyes the day of surgery, do not be alarmed. Most often, that ability will return within a few days. If too much upper eyelid skin was removed, the problem may persist. Treatment involves restoring skin to your eyelids through skin grafts. Although skin grafts may solve the functional problem, they may create a cosmetic problem because grafted skin is never a perfect match.

Corneal Abrasion

During surgery, you may sustain an inadvertent scratch to your cornea. A corneal abrasion is temporarily painful and is treated by patching the eye closed for one to three days. After healing, no lasting discomfort or visual disturbance will occur.

Skin Cysts

Tiny skin cysts, called milia, may appear along the scar line. This is more common when stitches remain for five or more days. Milia go away on their own or may be removed in the office as a minor procedure.

Abnormal Upper Lid Position

Correction of upper eyelid droop is tricky, and tiny displacements of the eyelids are obvious. Consequently, revision surgery is often needed. Following repair, both eyelids may be too high, both eyelids may be too low, or they may simply be uneven.

Telltale Signs

Unlike the telltale signs of a face-lift or a forehead lift, which cause only cosmetic problems, some telltale signs of eyelid surgery can alter eyelid function. These have already been discussed in the section on complications.

Lower Lid Retraction

If the lower eyelid falls below the iris, then the white of the eye will be visible. This is called lower lid retraction, or ectropion, and is considered a cosmetic problem (figure 4-9). It may also cause dry eye syndrome. The problem is most commonly due to a lax lower eyelid, but it may also be due

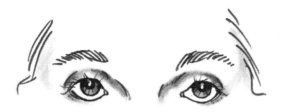

FIGURE 4-9: *Lower lid retraction is evident by the white of the eye below the iris. It may be caused by too much skin removal, lack of lower eyelid support, or both.*

to removal of too much skin. This is a difficult problem to solve. Treatment involves canthopexy (tightening the lower lid), skin grafting to the lower lid, or both.

Upper Lid Retraction

Upper lid retraction, also called lagophthalmos, is an inability to close the eye completely and is usually due to overzealous skin removal. Eventually, damage to the cornea will occur if the lid cannot protect it.

In order to correct this problem, a skin graft to the upper eyelid is required. Skin grafts never look the same as natural skin, and the final cosmetic result will unfortunately be less than satisfactory.

Hollow (Sunken) Eyes

If too much fat is removed, your eyes will appear sunken. Hollowness conjures images of malnutrition. This is one of the most common telltale signs of eyelid surgery and is unfortunately hard to correct.

Cost

In the United States, the range of total fees for eyelid surgery extends from $3,000 to $6,000. The average cost is:

Surgeon's fee	$ 3,000
Anesthesiologist's fee	$ 700
Operating room (facility) fee	$ 800
Total	$4,500

The Lower Eyelid

Retraction Versus Droop
In retraction, the lower eyelid is pulled downward due to previous surgery or trauma. In droop, the lower eyelid is pulled downward due to natural causes such as gravity or gradual loss of support as aging occurs. Lower eyelid droop is associated with severe lid laxity.

See "Fees" in Chapter 1 for various factors that might affect your own actual cost.

These averages are for removal of skin and/or fat from both upper and lower eyelids. If you need repair of droopy upper or lower lids, expect to pay more. If you are interested in skin and/or fat removal of either the upper or the lower lids, but not both, then plan to pay an average total fee of $3,000.

Duration of Results

Some women need eyelid surgery only once. Others may seek repeat eyelid surgery within a decade. Young women with puffy eyes who undergo fat removal may seek eyelid surgery again as they age.

Satisfaction

Eyelid surgery can rejuvenate old, droopy, tired eyes. Because the eyes are the focal points of the face, eyelid surgery can affect the whole appearance. The procedure and recovery are relatively brief. Satisfaction is generally high, and eyelid surgery is one of the three most commonly sought cosmetic procedures.

Questions to Ask Your Plastic Surgeon

Are my upper eyelids droopy?

Do I have adequate tone of my lower eyelid?

Do I need lower eyelid support?

Will the lower eyelid incision be inside or outside of the eyelid?

How do you avoid removing too much skin?

Am I at risk for dry eye syndrome?

Do I need a forehead lift, too?

Concluding Thoughts

Cosmetic eyelid problems may be a combination of excess skin, protruding fat, and eyelid position. Surgery should be closely tailored to the needs of the individual. As with any procedure, there are risks; but here, the stakes are high. Finding a well-qualified plastic surgeon together with your understanding of the issues, will give you the best chance for a safe and successful outcome.

Tips and Traps

If your surgeon tells you a forehead lift is also needed, avoid eyelid surgery alone if you want your final result to be optimal.

Dark circles under your eyes will not disappear after eyelid surgery unless you are able to make them disappear before surgery by stretching your lower eyelid skin.

Your crow's feet will not improve through eyelid surgery.

Vertical frown lines between your eyebrows will not improve following eyelid surgery.

Do not have a chemical peel or laser procedure within three months of lower eyelid surgery if the incisions are made on the outside of your eyelids.

If you do not need skin removed from your lower lids, then request an incision on the inside of your eyelids.

Eyelid surgery will not rejuvenate your skin. For that, pursue skin care or a resurfacing procedure described in Chapters 11 and 12.

If you have dry eyes, get evaluated by an ophthalmologist before surgery to identify correctable causes. Surgery can usually be performed; however, your surgeon should tighten your lower lid or remove less skin than initially planned, or else your dry eye symptoms may worsen.

If your lower eyelids fail the laxity tests, expect a lid tightening (procedure such as canthopexy) to prevent lower eyelid droop and dry eye syndrome. Beware a plastic surgeon who does not assess your lid tone or who does not recommend canthopexy if your lid tone is weak.

Understand that canthopexy causes more swelling and may delay recovery by an additional week.

Sleep in a recliner or with your head elevated on pillows for the first several days after surgery to minimize swelling. Apply ice frequently!

5

Refining Your Nose

Rhinoplasty

BETSY, *a 29-year-old computer programmer, was shy. She had difficulty meeting people, and was always the quiet one in the crowd. Whenever she met someone, she felt certain that they were staring at her nose, even when they were not. She knew that the problem was not in the way others saw her, but in how she saw herself. Her large nose distorted her self-image and made it difficult for her to be comfortable around others. After undergoing rhinoplasty, she immediately became confident, outgoing, and talkative. She felt better about herself and was therefore more comfortable around others. Within six months, she moved from the programming division to the sales division—something she had never even imagined.*

*I*ndisputably the nose is a pivotal facial feature. A nose in harmony with the rest of your face blends and is unnoticed. A nose in disharmony draws attention. Because the nose is a focal point, any minor unattractive feature may seem significant and can alter self-image.

Cosmetic nose surgery is known as *rhinoplasty*. The name is derived from the Greek "rhino" (meaning nose) and "plasty" (meaning to shape or reform). Rhinoplasty can change noses in many ways. It is possible to enlarge a small nose, reduce a large nose, smooth a bumpy nose, lift a droopy nose, straighten a crooked nose, narrow a wide nose, widen a narrow nose, shorten a long nose, lengthen a short nose, and so on. Yet, limitations exist. Your plastic surgeon will help you understand whether your goals are realistic and whether you are a good candidate.

Is There a Perfect Nose?

Every face is different in size, shape, and contour, and therefore the perfect nose for each face is different. Despite this, certain nasal characteristics are

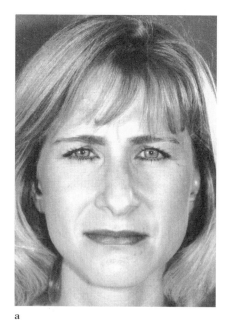

a

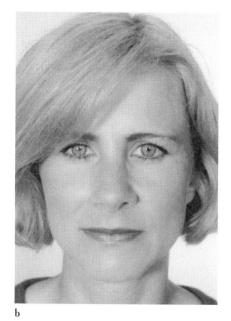

b

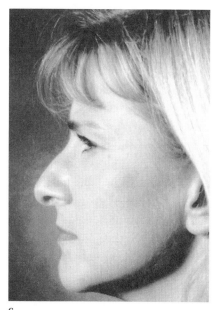

c

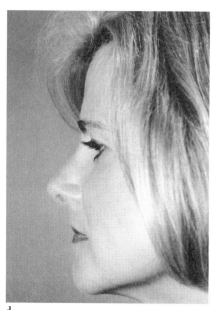

d

(a and c) Before rhinoplasty. (b and d) After rhinoplasty.

considered aesthetically pleasing for nearly everyone. When evaluating your nose critically, you and your surgeon should consider the following characteristics but not be confined by them. Some features of a cosmetically appealing nose are a straight nasal dorsum, a narrow nasal tip, a small dip between the nasal dorsum and the tip, an appropriate angle between the nostrils and upper lip, an appropriate amount of nasal projection from the face, and an appropriate width. Some surgeons will measure the angles of your nose to help formulate a surgical plan (fig. 5-1).

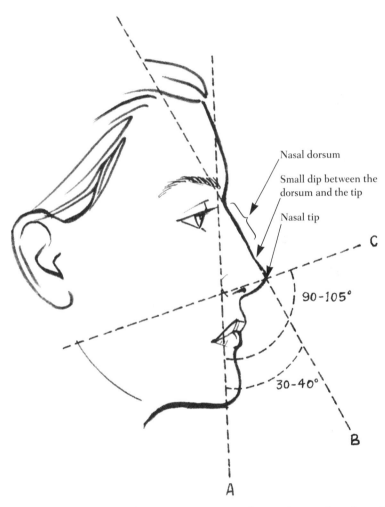

Nasal dorsum

Small dip between the dorsum and the tip

Nasal tip

C

90-105°

30-40°

B

A

FIGURE 5-1: *Evaluation of your nose. Your surgeon may study your photographs to determine the angles between your nose and face. For women, the ideal angle between lines A and B is 30–40°. If it is greater than 40°, then your nose is too prominent. If it is less than 30°, then your nose is too flat. Line C is through the base of the nose and reflects tip rotation. If it is greater than 105°, then your tip is upturned. If it is less than 90°, then your tip is too low.*

Nasal Asymmetry

Recognize your asymmetries before having any cosmetic surgery. After surgery, some asymmetries will be improved, whereas others will not. Everyone has a long side of the nose and a short side of the nose. Prior to surgery, you may fail to notice this in yourself. Afterward, it may become obvious, simply because you will study your nose more carefully. You may think it is because of the operation, but most likely it was present before surgery.

The Importance of Your Chin

Your chin plays a crucial role in the appearance of your nose (see Chapter 6). A weak chin can make an appropriately sized nose stand out. This problem should be solved by chin augmentation, not nose surgery.

NANCY, *a 31-year-old advertising executive, thought her nose was too big for her face. In reality, her problem was a weak chin. She accepted this when she saw her profile in a photograph. Moving her chin forward in the picture brought her whole profile into harmony. She underwent chin implant placement and was satisfied that her nose no longer appeared large.*

Is Rhinoplasty for You?

Not everyone is a good candidate for rhinoplasty. In order to have successful surgery, you must meet four criteria:

- You can describe specifically what bothers you
- You are young enough to adjust to your new nose
- You do not use nasal medications or drugs
- You accept that revision surgery may be needed

If you fail to meet any of these criteria, your chance for a satisfactory outcome will be much lower.

Describe Specifically What Bothers You

It is difficult for a surgeon if you simply say, "I want my nose to look better." Be specific about the changes you seek, and do not assume that the changes you desire are necessarily the changes your plastic surgeon would make without your input.

Before you see your plastic surgeon, spend time with your mirror. Decide which nasal features specifically bother you. Write them down so that you do

JANET, *a 34-year-old soccer mom, disliked her nose but was unable to express exactly which features bothered her. She simply wanted to "make it better." Her nasal tip was somewhat bulbous, and her nose was slightly wide and prominent. Yet, without her input, there was no way to know which specific features troubled her. I was unwilling to perform rhinoplasty without her guidance, so she found another surgeon. Several months later, she returned complaining that the other surgeon had ruined her nose, yet her nose appeared much improved. I pointed out that without her input, no surgeon could possibly know how to make her nose to her liking. She subsequently had at least one revision surgery by another surgeon and, not surprisingly, is still displeased.*

KAY, *a 46-year-old social worker, had always wanted rhinoplasty and was finally able to afford it. She knew exactly how she wanted her nose changed and was a good candidate for surgery. However, at her age, she was accustomed to her nose, despite her displeasure with its appearance. Because of this, she was at risk for dissatisfaction with her result. Knowing this, she still wished to proceed. Following rhinoplasty, her result closely matched her goal, but she was uncomfortable with her appearance. It took two years for her to finally accept her new nose, and she admitted that she had underestimated the difficulty of adjustment.*

not forget to mention each concern. The only way to ensure that your goals are aligned is through careful discussion.

Cosmetic nasal surgery results in specific structural changes in the nose. If you are unable to identify specific features of your nose that you dislike, it is unlikely that any change will result in satisfaction.

Be Young Enough to Adjust to Your New Nose

Younger women are better candidates for rhinoplasty than older women are. The older you are, the more slowly you will adapt to a change in your facial features. Younger patients (under 30) adapt more easily because their self-images are not as entrenched.

You become accustomed to your nose and facial characteristics over the course of your lifetime. By the time you reach your 50s, you will be so used to your facial features that any change in appearance, no matter how positive, is likely to leave you dissatisfied. Dissatisfaction arises because you will think you look like a different person.

This issue of adjustment applies to changes in bone, cartilage, and muscle that alter basic facial features. It does not usually apply to rejuvenation procedures such as eyelid surgery or forehead lift, because they do not typically affect the underlying structure of the face.

Use No Nasal Medications or Drugs

If you use nasal sprays, steroids, other nasal medications, or abuse cocaine, you will be at increased risk for bleeding and healing problems. A healing problem could result in a hole in your nasal septum that may require further surgery. You should stop using nasal medications for at least three months before surgery to ensure the safest outcome. If you abuse cocaine, then it is probably safe to assume that you have more problems than a potential hole in your nose. Regardless, do not seek any nasal surgery until after you have conquered your addiction, refrained from cocaine use for one year, and notified your surgeon of your previous abuse.

Accept That Revision Surgery May Be Needed

At least 20 percent of all women who have rhinoplasty will need a revision. The reasons are many. Perhaps the result appears unnatural. Perhaps the changes were inadequate. Perhaps the initial results were promising, but the nose changed unfavorably over subsequent months.

Operations on the nose are fraught with difficulty and unpredictability. Before you have your first rhinoplasty, you must accept the fact that at best there is a one in five chance that you will undergo reoperation.

Incisions and Scars

Your surgeon has two main options for rhinoplasty incisions: closed and open (see comparison Table 5-1).

Closed Rhinoplasty

In a closed rhinoplasty, all incisions are made inside the nose, so there are no visible scars. The surgeon has only a limited view of the cartilage and bone. Yet many plastic surgeons are comfortable with this technique and achieve excellent results.

Open Rhinoplasty

In open rhinoplasty, the nose skin is lifted, allowing the surgeon a clear view of the cartilage and bone. The surgeon makes a small incision on the underside of the nasal tip, between the two nostrils (fig. 5-2). Additional incisions are also made inside the nose. Some surgeons prefer this approach because it allows them greater visibility of some portions of the nose.

Three disadvantages of open rhinoplasty are (1) a scar between the nostrils, (2) significant postoperative swelling, and (3) decreased ability of your surgeon to judge the aesthetic results of changes as they are made during surgery. Although scars are permanent, they are often imperceptible once

TABLE 5–1. *Comparison of Closed and Open Rhinoplasty*

RHINOPLASTY TYPE	ADVANTAGES	DISADVANTAGES
Closed	*No scar outside the nose* *Less swelling (1–6 weeks)*	*May be difficult to correct* *some complex nasal problems*
Open	*Excellent view for surgeon*	*Small scar under the nose* *More swelling (1–6 months)*

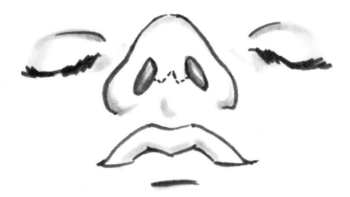

FIGURE 5-2: *Open rhinoplasty incision. An open rhinoplasty relies on a small incision between the nostrils. This incision usually heals imperceptibly. The bigger problem is swelling, which may take months to improve.*

they heal, but not always. Swelling following an open rhinoplasty lasts two to six months longer than after a closed rhinoplasty. With diligent use of ice and elevation, some are able to minimize the duration and degree of swelling.

Closed Versus Open

The closed procedure is probably sufficient for most patients and most surgeons. Open rhinoplasty is usually reserved for those with severely deformed noses, previous nasal operations, or particularly challenging problems. In these people, the need for open view of the cartilage during surgery outweighs the visible scars and persistent swelling after surgery.

Modifying What Forms Your Nose

The upper half of your nose is bone, and the lower half is cartilage. Rhinoplasty modifies the cartilage, bone, or both.

Bone

Modification of bone may involve reducing it, augmenting it, or refining it. If it is to be reduced, it often must be fractured and repositioned. If you have a hump on your nose, expect that your doctor will fracture your nose after removing the hump.

Women who seek revision surgery often require bone augmentation. This can be achieved through use of your own bone. Your surgeon can harvest bone from your skull, rib, or hipbone, which of course leaves you with another area of pain, healing, and scarring. Despite this temporary disadvantage, using your own bone lowers the risk of infection and is more stable than the alternative, namely, prosthetic material. Prosthetic material can be made from synthetic materials such as plastic polymers or naturally occurring materials such as cadaver bone (see Chapter 6). If your surgeon sees a need for bone augmentation, be certain you understand the plan.

Cartilage

Cartilage can be modified by reducing it, refining it, or augmenting it. Initial rhinoplasties usually involve reducing and refining the cartilage; revision rhinoplasties are more likely to require rebuilding with grafts or prosthetic material. Cartilage grafts may be harvested from your nose, your ear, or your rib. As with bone grafts, this will involve another incision. Synthetic material is rarely used for cartilage replacement.

Modifying Your Nasal Airway

In altering the appearance of your nose, rhinoplasty may or may not affect your nasal airway.

Improvement in Nasal Airway

Your nasal septum is on the inside of your nose and separates the left and right nasal passages. If your nasal septum is crooked, straightening it may improve your breathing. This surgical procedure is known as *septoplasty* and is performed through incisions on the inside of your nose. It does not alter appearance. It may be performed with or without rhinoplasty. If your crooked nasal septum is causing breathing problems, your insurance company may pay for this septoplasty. Neither septoplasty nor rhinoplasty will improve nasal obstruction due to allergies or nasal swelling.

Worsening of Your Nasal Airway

One potential complication of rhinoplasty is nasal obstruction. Loss of nasal support or over-narrowing of the nose may cause this. If this occurs, it can be improved through further surgery.

What to Expect

Rhinoplasty is commonly performed under sedation anesthesia, and you will be allowed to go home the same day. Discomfort is moderate and will be controlled with prescription pain medication. You will likely be presentable in public with makeup within one to two weeks.

Vital Statistics

Anesthesia: *Sedation or general.*

Location of operation: *Office or hospital.*

Length of surgery: *1–3 hours.*

Length of stay: *Outpatient (home same day).*

Discomfort: *Moderate. If your nasal bones are broken as part of the procedure, expect 5–10 days of prescription pain medication. If not, expect 2–7 days. Use a humidifier and nasal saline spray to keep your nasal passages moist and comfortable.*

Bruising: *Improves in 3–10 days if your nasal bones are not broken, and 7–14 days if they are. Black eyes are not unusual during this time.*

Swelling: *Improves in 1–6 weeks following closed rhinoplasty and 1–6 months following open. Sleeping in a recliner after surgery helps substantially. Applying ice for 2–4 days is also important.*

Numbness: *Numbness of the tip of your nose is expected and will last for several weeks.*

Bandages: *Your nose will be taped at the completion of surgery. If your nasal bones were broken, you will also receive a small cast. The cast and tape are removed in 5–10 days.*

Stitches: *You will have absorbable stitches on the inside of your nose. If your rhinoplasty was open, you will also have stitches under the tip of your nose. They will be removed in 4–7 days.*

Packing: *May be used to control bleeding. If so, it will be removed in 1–7 days. While packing is in place, it is uncomfortable. Removal is also unpleasant. This is probably the worst part of rhinoplasty.*

Makeup: *May be worn after the cast and tape have been removed.*

Presentable in public: *You will be presentable in 1–2 weeks, but you may need makeup to conceal your bruises. Swelling will last longer than bruising and may make you self-conscious, but it will not be an automatic telltale sign of rhinoplasty.*

Work: *You may feel capable of returning within a week, but your appearance will be the limiting factor.*

Exercise: *May be resumed in 3–4 weeks. Avoid contact sports for 6 weeks.*

Final result: *May be seen as soon as 3 months or as late as 2 years. The majority see their final result within 6 months.*

To help you to plan for and recover from your procedure, reread Steps 7 and 10 of chapter 1.

Complications

When your operation is performed by a qualified plastic surgeon, both your procedure and recovery will likely be uneventful. Even in ideal circumstances, however, complications may occur. In addition to the specific complications mentioned here, refer to Chapter 1 for general complications with any procedure.

Bleeding and Other Major Complications

Severe bleeding may occur during or after surgery, and nasal packing may be needed to control it. The risk of severe bleeding is less than 2 percent. Exceedingly rare but life-threatening problems associated with the brain can also occur—including leakage of cerebrospinal fluid (CSF), accumulation of air around the brain, meningitis, and even death. After all, the human brain and nose are separated by nothing more than a delicate bone, which may fracture from the forces delivered during rhinoplasty.

Sinusitis

A sinus infection may occur within weeks of rhinoplasty. If a sinus infection occurs, it is usually due to internal nasal swelling. Swelling temporarily obstructs the opening to the nasal passages that drains the sinuses, thereby triggering sinusitis. Symptoms include foul nasal drainage, facial pain, headaches, and fevers. If you have any of these symptoms, contact your plastic surgeon immediately. A combination of antibiotics, nasal sprays, and decongestant pills will improve symptoms and keep your sinuses healthy until swelling improves.

Bumpy Nose

If you have thin skin, you will easily feel any irregularities of your underlying cartilage or bone. These irregularities require additional surgery to smooth out the nose.

When Can I Stop Worrying About Complications?

Most complications occur within a predictable time following surgery. If you do not develop them within the time periods noted, you can fairly conclude that you are probably free of these complications:

TIME SINCE SURGERY	POSSIBLE COMPLICATION
2 weeks	*Severe problems such as meningitis or CSF leakage*
3 weeks	*Sinusitis*
3 months	*Bumpy nose*
3 months	*Nasal obstruction*

Implant extrusion, however, may occur at any time. If you have synthetic implants, you can never conclude that you are free of complications.

Nasal Obstruction

Rhinoplasty can obstruct your nasal breathing, even if you had no previous breathing problems. This may be due to collapse of cartilage or over-narrowing of nasal bones. Most breathing problems can be improved through further surgery.

Implant Extrusion

If synthetic material was used to augment your nasal bones or cartilage, it may eventually wear through the skin or through the lining of your nose. If the implanted material extrudes, it must be removed. Later you will need another operation to reconstruct your nose. Synthetic material should not be used again. Your own cartilage or bone should be used because they will not extrude after healing.

Telltale Signs

Scooped Out Nose

Also called ski slope nose, a scooped out nose can occur if too much bone and cartilage was removed during surgery (fig. 5-3a). This appears unnatural and can be corrected by placing a cartilage graft, bone graft, or synthetic implant into your nose.

Polly Beak

A polly beak, or parrot beak, is another telltale (fig. 5-3b). It may not be evident for a year or more after surgery, and correction requires revision rhinoplasty.

Pug Nose

A pug nose is an upturned nose that is unattractive and unnatural (fig. 5-3c). This is due to over-shortening of the nose and may be corrected through revision rhinoplasty with cartilage grafts.

Pinched Tip

If your surgeon removes too much cartilage near the rim of your nostrils, the tip of your nose may appear pinched, notched, or collapsed (fig. 5-3d). This may be corrected by placing cartilage grafts during revision surgery.

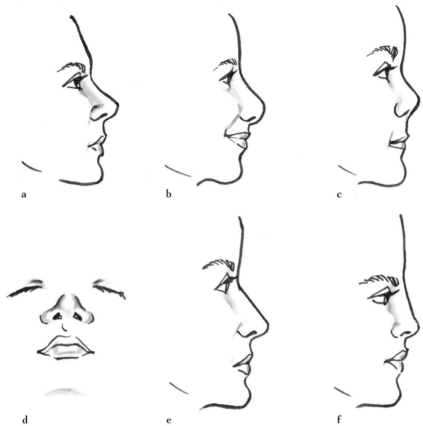

FIGURE 5-3: *Telltale signs. (a) scooped out nose; (b) polly beak; (c) pug nose; (d) pinched tip; (e) straight nose; (f) nose that starts too high.*

Straight Nose

If your nose appears perfectly straight in profile, it will look unnatural (fig. 5-3e). Natural noses may appear relatively straight, but they usually have a small dip just above the tip of the nose (fig. 5-1). Perfectly straight noses are most likely to occur after placement of a synthetic implant and can be modified through additional surgery.

Nose Starts Too Low or Too High

If you look at your own nose in profile, you will see that your nose begins at the level of your upper eyelashes. If your nasal dorsum has been overzealously lowered, your nose may appear to start too low on your face. Alternatively, if your nasal dorsum has been built up with a graft or implant, it can appear that your nose starts too high on your face (fig. 5-3f). Both of these problems can be corrected through revision rhinoplasty. Interestingly, in some parts of the world, a high nose is considered attractive.

Cost

In the United States, the range of total fees for rhinoplasty extends from $3,500 to $6,500. (In the New York City area, the range is $6,000 to $12,000.) The average cost is:

Surgeon's fee	$3,500
Anesthesiologist's fee	$ 700
Operating room (facility) fee	$ 800
Total	**$5,000**

See "Fees" in Chapter 1 for various factors that might affect your own actual cost.

The Final Result

Because natural forces continue to act on your nose after surgery, your final result may not be evident for one to two years. You may be pleased with your early result once the swelling has improved, but this is not a guarantee that you will be ultimately satisfied. If you are pleased with your results after two years, then you will likely remain satisfied.

Duration of Results

If you are satisfied with the final results after your first rhinoplasty, then you should never need another one.

Satisfaction

Rhinoplasty is a powerful operation. When it achieves the desired results, satisfaction is immense. A successful rhinoplasty can change one's personality from shy and withdrawn to exuberant and outgoing. When rhinoplasty yields an undesirable result, however, dissatisfaction is equally great. When considering rhinoplasty, you must consider these factors together. There is an 80 percent chance that you will be satisfied, and possibly elated; but there is a 20 percent chance that you will be significantly dissatisfied.

Revision Rhinoplasty

At least 20 percent of people who have rhinoplasty seek revision. If you are dissatisfied with the appearance of your nose following rhinoplasty, this does not necessarily mean that your plastic surgeon performed poorly. If your surgeon agrees that your result is unsatisfactory, agrees that your expectations are realistic, has a specific plan for correcting the problem, and has experience in revision rhinoplasty, you should allow him or her to reoperate. Understand, however, that each procedure on your nose will be much more difficult than the one before. Furthermore, revision surgery is not guaranteed to solve your problem. For the best results in revision rhinoplasty, find a surgeon who is skilled in rhinoplasty as well as revision rhinoplasty—two entirely different operations.

To minimize your need for revision rhinoplasty, seek an experienced surgeon. Look for one who has performed at least one hundred rhinoplasties over at least 10 years. The exact number per year is not as relevant as the doctor's overall experience, which builds over time. The time frame is important, as final results in rhinoplasty may not be evident for two years. As such, surgeons must have the opportunity to assess their own results over time as they modify their techniques. Plastic surgeons who continue to perform rhinoplasties after having performed 100 over 10 years likely do so because of satisfactory results. Those who have unsatisfactory results often abandon this operation before 10 years has passed. Plastic surgeons, like most people, enjoy success and avoid failure.

Yet *even in the most experienced hands*, the revision rate is 20 percent. If you do require revision, wait at least one year following your first operation. Because the appearance of your nose may change over time, the need for revision rhinoplasty may not be evident even for two years. Find out how long your surgeon's policy concerning revision rhinoplasty applies.

> ## Questions to Ask Your Plastic Surgeon
>
> *How many rhinoplasties have you performed?*
>
> *How long have you been performing rhinoplasties?*
>
> *Can you improve my breathing through surgery?*
>
> *Do you plan to do open or closed rhinoplasty?*
>
> *Will you use synthetic material?*
>
> *Will I have nasal packing?*
>
> *What is your policy regarding revision surgery, and how long does it apply?*

Tips and Traps

Know exactly what you want changed and how you want it changed before you see your plastic surgeon. Make a list.

Make sure that you and your plastic surgeon have a clear understanding of the planned changes.

Avoid a surgeon who downplays the difficulty of nasal surgery.

Make sure you and your surgeon examine your chin before surgery. If your surgeon recommends chin implant instead of or in addition to rhinoplasty, listen to that advice.

The older you are, the more difficult it will be for you to adjust to your new nose. Consider this carefully if you are over 40.

Understand that there is at least a 20 percent chance you will need revision surgery.

Asking your surgeon's revision rate is of little help because many women seek revision from a different surgeon. Your surgeon may not know how many patients have had a second operation.

Avoid all nasal medications for three months before surgery.

For the first two weeks following surgery, use a humidifier and nasal saline spray to keep your nasal passages moist and comfortable.

Sleep in a recliner or with your head elevated on pillows for the first several days to minimize swelling. Apply ice frequently!

If you require revision surgery, wait at least one year after your last nasal operation.

Concluding Thoughts

Rhinoplasty modifies the bone and cartilage of your nose to effect a change in appearance. The operation is tailored to the specific needs of the individual. This is the most difficult cosmetic procedure performed by plastic surgeons. It is critical that you find a plastic surgeon who is highly experienced in this procedure. Cosmetic nose surgery has the potential to create a new appearance and lend new confidence. Just be careful.

6

Bringing Out Your Chin and Cheeks

Facial Implants

*F*acial implants for the chin and cheeks are cosmetic surgical options that are often overlooked. Chin and cheek implants may create a stronger appearance and bring harmony to your face. A properly chosen chin implant can even enhance the appearance of your nose.

GAIL, *a 39-year-old nurse anesthetist, was self-conscious of her facial contour and profile. Because she did not like the idea of having a synthetic material in her body, she pursued rhinoplasty and neck liposuction, both of which offered some improvement but failed to give her the look she wanted. When she finally underwent chin and cheek augmentation, she achieved the appearance she desired with full, high cheeks and a strong chin.*

Unfortunately, facial implants are not risk free. Because implant procedures involve placement of different materials, you must carefully examine all implant options. Your understanding of the implant materials available is key to getting the best outcome, reducing your risk, and having a lasting result.

Chin and cheek implants, although similar in many respects, differ in three important ways: why people choose to have them, how they are placed, and what might be done instead. After exploring these notable differences, this chapter will focus on the recovery period, costs, risks, and implant options, all of which are similar for chin and cheek implants.

If you are interested only in cheek implants, skip to the next section.

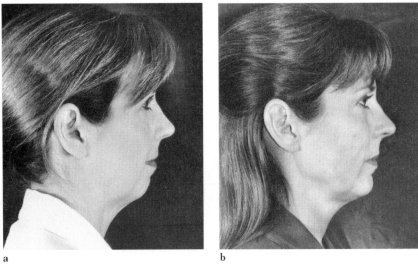

a   b

(a) Before chin augmentation. (b) After chin augmentation.

Chin Implants

Reasons for Chin Augmentation

Together, your chin and nose determine your profile. Look at your profile by using a handheld mirror in conjunction with a wall mirror. Imagine a straight line drawn from your forehead through the forwardmost point of your upper lip. In your mind, extend this line down to the level of your chin (fig. 6-1). If

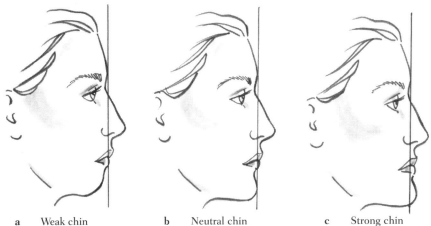

    a   Weak chin   **b**   Neutral chin   **c**   Strong chin

FIGURE 6-1: *The effect of chin projection. All noses in this illustration are the same size, but they look different. (a) A weak chin that falls behind the vertical line of the face causes the nose to look large. (b) A neutral chin. (c) An overprojected chin causes the nose to look flat. Chin augmentation commonly brings a weak chin into neutral position and can make a large nose look more proportionate.*

PATTI, *a 41-year-old pilot, was generally happy with her facial features but disliked her small chin; she did not think it matched her assertive personality. To hide her profile, she wore her hair long and forward. After much thought, she underwent chin augmentation. Following surgery, she changed her hairstyle to reveal her profile.*

your chin meets the imaginary line, then you have sufficient chin projection. If your chin extends beyond this line, then you have a strong chin. If your chin falls short of this line, then your chin is underprojected. To see this more clearly, have someone take a photograph of your profile and use a ruler to draw the line.

A weak chin can make an average-sized nose appear large. Strengthening the chin through chin augmentation can bring the entire profile into harmony. In figure 6-1, all noses are the same size. However, in the illustration with a weak chin, the nose appears larger. If your surgeon suggests chin augmentation instead of or in addition to rhinoplasty, seriously consider this advice. A chin implant may have a positive impact on your entire facial appearance.

Details of Chin Implant Surgery

Chin implantation involves placing a prosthetic material in front of your chin bone (fig. 6-2). Incisions can either be made under your chin or inside your mouth (fig. 6-3). Both are reasonable options. An incision in your mouth avoids a visible scar, but an incision under your chin usually goes without notice. Most surgeons place chin implants through the mouth, unless they are performing a face-lift. A face-lift usually requires a chin incision, so the same incision can be used to place the implant.

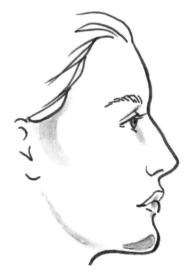
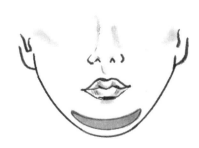

FIGURE 6-2: *Position of chin implant.*

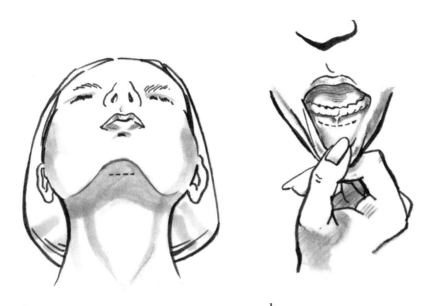

a   b

FIGURE 6-3: *(a) Incision under the chin. (b) Incision inside the mouth.*

Chin Augmentation Without an Implant

It is possible to augment your chin by sliding a portion of your chin bone forward (fig. 6-4). This is known as *genioplasty* and involves surgically cutting your chin bone, moving it forward, and securing it with screws or wires.

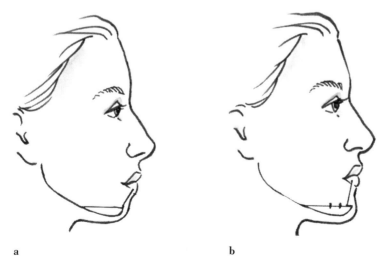

a   b

FIGURE 6-4: *Chin augmentation without an implant. (a) The chin before surgery. A solid line depicts where the bone will be cut. (b) The chin in its new position with the resultant strengthening of profile. The two small vertical marks indicate wires holding the bone in its new position.*

Genioplasty offers the advantage of using your own bone and hence yields lower rates of infection, extrusion, erosion, and migration (see "Complications"). The disadvantages are slightly longer procedure time and recovery. Further, genioplasty is more difficult to modify than chin implantation. If you are displeased with your result, the bone will need to be re-broken and moved again. According to the American Society of Plastic and Reconstructive Surgeons, the average total cost for genioplasty is a few hundred dollars more than implant surgery.

If you are not interested in cheek implants, then skip ahead to "Considerations in Common."

Cheek Implants

Reasons for Cheek Augmentation

Most people consider prominent cheekbones to be attractive, as evidenced by the facial features of successful professional models. Women who have low or flat cheekbones may seek cheek augmentation to achieve this aesthetic ideal. Because most women who seek cosmetic surgery have other aesthetic priorities, this operation is not as common as some other procedures. Yet, when women do choose to pursue cheek augmentation, they are usually rewarded.

Details of Cheek Augmentation Surgery

Cheek augmentation involves placement of prosthetic material in front of your cheekbones to create the appearance of full, high cheeks (fig. 6-5). The incisions for cheek augmentation are almost always made inside your mouth between the cheeks and gums. These scars are never visible. Other options for the incisions are in your lower eyelids or in front of your ears. These incisions are usually considered only if eyelid surgery or face-lift are performed at the same time.

Cheek Augmentation Without an Implant

Unlike the chin bone, which can be fractured and moved forward for augmentation, the cheekbones do not lend themselves to such a procedure. If you are emphatic about using your own bone for cheek augmentation, a portion of your skull, rib, or hip bone can be used as a graft. The disadvantages of bone grafts are that they must be harvested from separate sites and may shrink after they have been placed. For purely cosmetic cheek augmentation, most surgeons use only implant material.

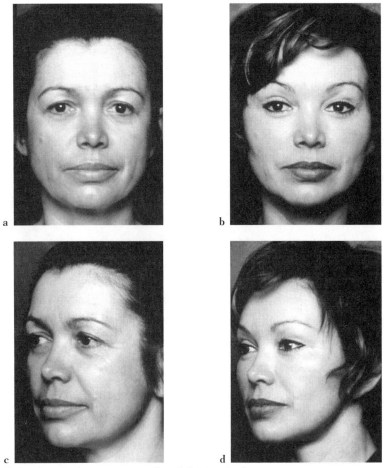

(a and c) Before cheek augmentation. (b and d) After cheek augmentation.

Edward O. Terino, M.D.

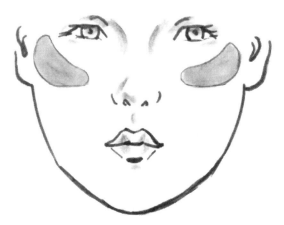

FIGURE 6-5: *Position of cheek implants.*

There is an exception to this rule. If you are having a face-lift at the same time, your surgeon may use extra facial tissue, called SMAS, to augment your cheeks. SMAS is a fibrous sheet of tissue located under the skin. It is pulled upward during two-layered face-lifts, and the excess is usually discarded. Instead of discarding the extra SMAS, some surgeons use it to create fullness in the cheek area. This technique arose in the mid-1990s, and some plastic surgeons report success with it. However, because SMAS is soft tissue, it may thin or droop with time. We may not know the long-term results for decades. Even if SMAS augmentation does not prove lasting, it is unlikely to cause problems. Therefore, if your surgeon recommends it and has had success with it, you should consider agreeing.

Considerations in Common

The rest of this chapter discusses issues that are common to both chin and cheek implants.

Adjusting to Your Implants

Placement of facial implants, like most cosmetic surgery procedures, has a positive impact on self-image of the recipient. However, with facial implants, there is a limit. The older the recipient is at the time of surgery, the less likely she will be pleased with her new facial structure. Over the years, we become accustomed to our basic facial features. Beyond a certain age, any change, no matter how attractive, may be unacceptable because it appears different. Women under 30 usually have no problem adapting. Those over 50 have problems adapting and may never become accustomed to their new appearance. Women from 30 to 50 have variable reactions.

Preexisting Asymmetry

Most people have asymmetric facial bones. Minor unevenness is common and usually goes unnoticed. Moderate or severe asymmetry, however, can be troublesome. If your chin or cheekbones are visibly uneven, they can be balanced through implant surgery. Your implants may be variably shaped, trimmed, and carved to achieve the desired contour and offset pre-existing asymmetry. Discuss this with your surgeon.

Timing for Surgery

Chin and cheek augmentation may be performed once the facial bones are fully developed, which is after the age of 15 for women.

What to Expect

Chin and cheek implants are commonly performed under sedation anesthesia, and you will be allowed to go home the same day. Discomfort is mild to moderate and will be controlled with prescription pain medication. You will be presentable in public within two weeks. Your final result will be evident within two months.

To help you plan for and recover from your procedure, reread Steps 7 and 10 of Chapter 1.

Complications

When your operation is performed by a qualified plastic surgeon, both your procedure and recovery will likely be uneventful. Even in ideal circumstances, however, complications may occur. In addition to the specific complications mentioned here, refer to Chapter 1 for general complications with any procedure.

Hematoma or Seroma

Immediately following surgery, you may develop a collection of blood or fluid around your implant. Small fluid collections will improve spontaneously, but larger collections often require surgery. Hematomas and seromas also increase the risk of infection and may affect your final result. Either risk is less than 1 percent.

Sensory Changes

Temporary numbness, pain, and tingling of the chin and cheeks are common and sensation usually normalizes within two to six weeks. Permanent numbness of the chin or cheeks can occur if the nerve was severely injured or cut during surgery.

You may develop delayed numbness several years following surgery if your implant shifts and presses on a nerve. Delayed numbness may be improved by removal of the implant. Following removal, you will return to your initial appearance. If you wish to have

Vital Statistics

Anesthesia: Sedation or general.

Location of operation: Office or hospital.

Length of surgery: 30 minutes for chin implant, 45–60 minutes for cheek implants.

Length of stay: Outpatient (home same day).

Discomfort: Mild to moderate. Anticipate 2–7 days of prescription pain medication.

Bruising: Uncommon.

Swelling: Lasts 1–2 weeks following chin implant and 2–3 weeks following cheek implants. Reduce swelling through constant head elevation and frequent application of ice.

Bandages: If any were placed, they will be removed in 1–5 days.

Stitches: If the incisions are inside your mouth, then absorbable stitches will be used and do not require removal. If skin incisions are used, stitches will be removed in 5 days.

Makeup: May be worn the day after surgery.

Presentable in public: You will be presentable in 2–5 days.

Work: You may feel capable of returning within 2–5 days, but your swelling will be the limiting factor.

Exercise: May be resumed in 2 weeks.

Final result: Will be seen between one and two months.

another implant placed, an alternative implant type may be selected that poses a lower risk of migration and impingement on your nerves.

Infection

The risk of infection is related to the type of implant used. Infection may initially be treated with oral or intravenous antibiotics, but implant removal is often necessary. Six months after the infection is cured, another implant may be placed. You and your surgeon will hopefully choose an implant material that poses a lower rate of infection than your first. (See "Implant Options" later in this chapter.)

Asymmetry

Asymmetry of the chin or cheeks may occur following surgery if implants are not placed symmetrically, if implants move out of position, or if pre-existing asymmetries are not identified and addressed properly. Postoperative asymmetry may be improved through additional surgery to modify the implants. Some implant materials are easier to modify than others, as described later in this chapter.

Implant Displacement

Migration or displacement of implants may occur, resulting in unnatural appearing chin or cheeks. Correction of this problem requires surgery to reposition the implant. Some implant materials are more prone to migration, as explained later in this chapter.

When Can I Stop Worrying About Complications?

As long as your implant is in place, you may never assume that you are clear of complications. Sensory changes, infection, implant displacement, bone erosion, implant detection, and need for further surgery may all occur months or years following placement of your implant.

Bone Erosion

Occasionally, an implant can become mobile. It may stay in its position, but can move by a fraction of an inch in all directions. When an implant becomes mobile, it generates friction with the underlying bone, which may in turn cause the bone to be slowly eaten away, or eroded. Chin erosion can be so significant that tooth roots are affected.

Some implant materials are more prone than others to move and to erode bone. Minor bone erosion is not unusual for some implants, but erosion down to tooth roots is exceedingly rare and mandates removal of the implant. Once the implant has been removed, further problems are unusual. Later, your surgeon may place a new implant, made of a material less likely to cause erosion.

Detecting the Implant Through Your Skin

You may be able to feel your implant through the skin, depending on the type of implant and its mobility. This is not necessarily a problem. If you are bothered by it, you may choose to have surgery to replace your implant with one that is less likely to move.

Extrusion of Implant

Some implants, particularly those that do not become attached to underlying bone, may erode your skin or the lining of your mouth. The implant may then become exposed, greatly increasing the risk of infection. Treatment usually involves removal of the implant. Once the wound heals, your surgeon may place a new implant. The new implant should be capable of adhering to your bone.

> **TERRY**, *a 47-year-old sales manager, had undergone chin implant placement eight years earlier by another surgeon. She was initially pleased, but as she aged, her skin thinned and her implant no longer looked natural. It appeared as a small round knob. Her chin no longer flowed with her jawline. Correction of her button chin involved removing her small implant and placing a longer one, resulting in a natural appearance.*

Need for Further Surgery

If you choose to get an implant, you should expect possible future operations. (This applies not only to plastic surgery implants, but also to artificial joints, pacemakers, and heart valves.) Implants are artificial devices; some may last a lifetime, others will not.

Telltale Signs

Witch's Chin

Witch's chin is droopy chin skin due to disruption of the attachments between skin and bone during surgery (fig. 6-6). Attempts to correct this problem through more surgery may not be successful. Plastic surgeons strive to avoid this difficult problem.

Button Chin

An unnaturally small or round chin may result if the implant is too small or narrow. This problem can be avoided by using a longer, broader implant that extends along the sides of your jaw. Correction of button chin requires surgery to exchange the implant for a longer one.

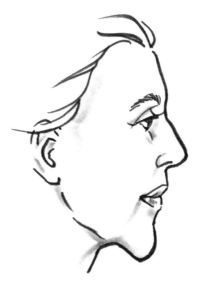

FIGURE 6-6: *Witch's chin. This problem is due to droopy skin and is difficult to correct through further surgery.*

Cost

In the United States, the range of total fees extends from $2,000 to $4,000 for chin implants and $3,500 to $5,000 for cheek implants. The average cost is:

	CHIN	CHEEKS
Surgeon's fee	$ 1,500	$ 2,200
Anesthesiologist's fee	$ 500	$ 600
Operating room (facility) fee	$ 600	$ 800
Implant fee	$ 400	$ 600
Total	$3,000	$4,200

See "Fees" in Chapter 1 for various factors that might affect your own actual cost.

The implant price quoted here reflects the marked-up price. Implants cost between $175 and $1,000 from the manufacturer. (Manufacturer prices are included in the table in the next section.) Your surgeon or the operating facility will mark up that price to cover the cost of ordering, shipping, and stocking implants.

If you are charged more than a 20 percent markup, you should question the price. Unfortunately, only plastic surgeons and hospitals may purchase implants, so you will be limited in your ability to negotiate.

Implant Options

Facial implants are made of several different materials. These materials vary in texture, consistency, firmness, and appearance. Each material has benefits and drawbacks; and each poses certain risks, including infection, asymmetry, displacement, bone erosion, and extrusion. Most surgeons prefer certain implants based on their experiences. (See Table 6-1 for a summary of material properties.)

Silastic

A flexible white or clear plastic, *Silastic* has been used for decades in pacemakers, artificial joints, and other medical prostheses. It is available in a wide range of sizes and shapes and is relatively inexpensive. It is easily placed and easily removed. The rate of infection is low. Implants that extend along the side of the chin are easily placed. For these reasons, silastic was the most commonly used implant for chin and cheek augmentation in the 1980s and early 1990s.

Silastic implants also pose some disadvantages. They do not attach to bone and may therefore move out of position after placement or erode underlying bone. And you may be able to feel the edges of the implant through your skin.

Hydroxyapatite

A strong, light, ceramic material, *hydroxyapatite* may be placed as multiple small granules or as a single large piece. The granules resemble tiny pebbles and require a smaller incision. Once placed, they can be molded for several days. The single piece requires a larger incision but will not migrate, as the granules may within the first few days.

Hydroxyapatite is porous like sea coral. This feature allows in-growth of tissue, bone, and blood vessels. In-growth anchors the implant and prevents it from migrating, extruding, becoming infected, or eroding

Overview of Implant Materials

- Silastic *is flexible white or clear plastic.*

- Hydroxyapatite *is a ceramic that resembles sea coral.*

- Polyethylene *is a type of plastic that also resembles sea coral.*

- Gore-Tex *is the same material used in high-quality raincoats.*

- Cadaver bone *is bone from deceased human donors.*

- Proplast *is a pliable plastic that resembles chewing gum.*

TABLE 6-1. *Comparison of Chin and Cheek Implant Materials*

	GENIOPLASTY (CHIN)	SILASTIC	HYDROXY-APATITE	POLY-ETHYLENE	GORE-TEX	CADAVER BONE	PROPLAST
RISK OF INFECTION	Rare	Low	Rare	Rare	Low	Rare	High
RISK OF BONE EROSION	None	Low	Rare	Rare	Rare	Rare	Moderate
RISK OF MIGRATION OR EXTRUSION	Rare	Low	Rare	Rare	Low	Rare	Moderate
RISK OF CONTRACTING INFECTION FROM THE IMPLANT	None	None	None	None	None	Theoretical	None
COST OF CHIN IMPLANT FROM THE MANUFACTURER	N/A	$175	$550	$225	$250	$1,000	N/A
COST OF TWO CHEEK IMPLANTS FROM THE MANUFACTURER	N/A	$225	$800	$400	$350	$1,200	N/A

N/A = Not applicable

underlying bone. This material may be shaped before placement to correct for preexisting asymmetries. And its shape is easy to revise through further surgery.

Polyethylene

Polyethylene is a plastic polymer that comes in single large pieces. Like hydroxyapatite, it resembles sea coral and has the same advantages as that implant material.

Gore-Tex

Gore-Tex is a cross between cloth and rubber. Its most common medical uses are for replacement arteries in bypass surgery of the legs and for reinforcement of hernia repairs. More than three million people in the United States have carried Gore-Tex in their bodies. The technical name for this material is expanded poly-tetra-fluoro-ethylene (ePTFE).

Gore-Tex is soft, pliable, porous, and may adhere to surrounding soft tissues. Because it does not attach to bone, it can migrate, become infected, and cause erosion. It is easily modified prior to placement but difficult to modify once in place. The infection and extrusion rates are low if the implant is not near the incision line. But near the incision line, infection and extrusion may occur and pose significant problems.

Cadaver Bone

Cadaver bone is human bone, obtained from donors shortly after death. After being freeze-dried and processed, it can be used for implants without being rejected. Cadaver bone has many advantages. It adheres to your own bone, and your own bone may even grow to replace it. So the implant is stable, resistant to motion, and resistant to infection. It does not erode your bone. It rarely extrudes or erodes through the skin or mucous membranes. And its shape is easy to modify later through another operation.

Cadaver bone may become variably absorbed, depending on its preparation. Some cadaver bone suppliers provide a reliable implant that will maintain most of its volume after placement. Poorly prepared cadaver bone, however, may shrink to a fraction of its size after it has been placed. If your surgeon recommends cadaver bone, ask about her long-term results.

Cadaver bone has at least two drawbacks. One is its high cost. The other is the risk of transmitting infections from the donor to the recipient. However, this risk appears to be only theoretical, because the donor's blood is tested and processed to eliminate potential infections. There have been no reports of transmitted infection from freeze-dried cadaver bone. (Fresh-frozen cadaver bone, unlike freeze-dried bone, does pose a possible risk of infection and is therefore not recommended.)

Finally, many women object to the notion of cadaver bone being placed in their bodies. For this reason alone, it is among the least popular implant materials used in cosmetic facial augmentation.

Proplast

Proplast is like plastic chewing gum. At one time, it was the most popular implant for facial augmentation. But Proplast caused so many complications that it was withdrawn from the market. The edges of Proplast implants curled and became evident through the skin of the face and the lining of the mouth, causing

---

Tissues from Deceased Donors

Bone and some collagen-related substances, such as Dermalogen and Alloderm (described in Chapters 11 and 13 respectively), are obtained from deceased donors. These materials are prepared via the same procedures and standards as for donor organs such as kidneys and hearts. Many donors are otherwise healthy young people who die in accidents. Before tissue is procured, each donor is tested for illness and infection, such as HIV. *The tissue banks that obtain and process these materials and organs follow the federally mandated tissue recovery guidelines and those of the American Association of Tissue Banks.*

According to the Musculoskeletal Transplant Foundation (the largest tissue bank for bone, ligaments, and tendons in the United States), your estimated odds of contracting the HIV *virus from cadaver collagen or bone is less than one in one and one-half million. Your chances of dying from falling out of bed are three times higher.*

skin to become red, irritated, and painful. It caused infections long after it was placed and it had to be removed when it became exposed or infected. However, this was difficult due to Proplast's dense adherence to surrounding tissues.

If you already have a Proplast implant, promptly seek the attention of a plastic surgeon if you develop redness or pain in the area of your implant. If your surgeon recommends a Proplast implant, refuse it. (Some surgeons stock implant materials for years and may therefore have Proplast available.)

Questions to Ask Your Plastic Surgeon

Can you correct my facial asymmetry?

Where will the incisions be?

Which implant material do you recommend and why?

Is the implant material associated with bone erosion?

How easy will it be to remove the implant, if needed?

Who pays for implant removal?

Tips and Traps

Each implant material offers certain advantages. Surgeons recommend the type of implant they think is most appropriate. Make sure you understand the disadvantages of each implant material.

Do not allow your surgeon to place a Proplast implant.

The older you are, the more difficult it will be for you to adapt to chin and cheek augmentation.

Anticipate the possible need for future surgery when accepting placement of any type of implant.

Duration of Results

Once your implant is in place, the results are usually lasting. Unless you develop complications, further surgery will not be necessary.

Satisfaction

The simplicity with which facial implants can be placed and the magnitude of change they can effect have contributed to their popularity. If you have no complications from your implant, then you will likely be satisfied with your result. If you develop complications, you may become rapidly disenchanted with your implant.

Concluding Thoughts

The perfect implant would be inexpensive, easy to place, easy to modify, and easy to remove. It would correct asymmetry, stay solidly in place, and be impossible to feel through the skin. It would never cause infection, never extrude, and never erode bone. Unfortunately, the perfect implant does not exist. Currently available implants, although imperfect, do provide safe, aesthetic augmentation with relatively few problems.

7

Enlarging Your Breasts

Breast Augmentation

*I*f you are like many women seeking breast augmentation, you are probably a well-educated professional who has been considering this operation for years. By now, you realize that the media scare surrounding breast implants was just that. But you still do not take the decision to proceed lightly. You, like most women, simply wish to have natural appearing breasts that bring your upper torso into harmony with the rest of your body. Not surprisingly, breast augmentation is the second most common cosmetic procedure in the United States.

When women seek breast augmentation, several questions are immediately raised:

- What materials are used in current breast implants?
- What was the truth about the silicone gel implant controversy?
- Can extra abdominal fat somehow be moved to the breasts for augmentation?
- Can fat be liposuctioned from the thighs and injected into the breasts?

The beginning of this chapter will address these questions, and the remainder will focus on breast augmentation with saline implants.

SONYA, *a 35-year-old gynecologist, chose her food carefully and worked out four times a week. Her body was trim and shapely, with the exception of her breasts. This was one thing that proper diet and exercise could not fix. She simply wanted her breasts to be in proportion with the rest of her body. Following breast augmentation, she felt balanced for the first time. She found to her surprise that she even stood straighter. Her only regret was that she did not have surgery sooner.*

Breast Implant Materials

Breast implants are similar to water balloons. The shell of the "balloon" is made of a durable, pliable plastic called solid silicone. (Solid silicone, or silastic, has been implanted in millions of people as pacemakers, artificial joints, heart valves, penile implants, and artificial lenses for the eye. Solid silicone is a very different substance than silicone gel, which filled silicone gel implants.)

Saline Versus Silicone Gel

For saline implants, the shell is filled with sterile salt water; for silicone gel implants, the shell is filled with silicone gel, which has the consistency of molasses. Silicone gel is superior to saline in appearance and feel. Whereas saline implants confer a stiff feeling to the breasts, silicone gel implants confer a softer and more pliable feeling. Silicone gel implants also move and hang more naturally, provided there is no capsular contracture (explained later). Finally, saline implants are heavier than a same-sized silicone gel implant.

AVAILABLE IMPLANTS

Since 1992, the only breast implants used in the United States for cosmetic augmentation have been saline. Saline implants have been used since the 1960s and are thought to be safe. Several studies conducted in the late 1990s support that conclusion.

THE FACTS ABOUT SILICONE GEL

From 1963 to 1992, millions of women received silicone gel implants. In the early 1990s, reports that leaking silicone gel implants caused connective tissue diseases (CTDs) appeared in the mass media without scientific verification. In response, the FDA restricted the use of silicone gel breast implants in 1992. Subsequently, litigation was successfully brought against Dow Corning, the largest manufacturer of silicone gel implants. Multitudes of healthy women understandably became alarmed and sought removal of their silicone gel implants. The tragedy was that the allegations against silicone gel implants were unfounded. They have never been shown to cause CTDs. Rather, numerous studies show that silicone gel implants neither cause nor contribute to CTDs. Whereas it is true that women with silicone gel implants do get CTDs, so do women without implants. Their risk of getting CTDs is the same.

DENISE, a 45-year-old flight attendant, had undergone breast augmentation at the age of 25. Although pleased with her results for 20 years, she sought to have her implants removed. The implants were causing no problems, but the fact that they were silicone gel implants greatly distressed her. She had been convinced through media reports that they posed a major risk to her health. It took three visits, several hours of discussion, and reams of scientific documentation to convince her that the charges against the silicone gel implants were unfounded.

Connective Tissue Diseases (CTDs)

Connective tissue diseases (CTDs) are autoimmune diseases in which the body's own defense system is triggered to identify normal body tissue as foreign and thereby attack it. Joints become stiff, skin develops rashes, muscles ache, and the body tires easily. Examples of CTDs include rheumatoid arthritis, lupus, scleroderma, fibromyalgia, and chronic fatigue syndrome. To date no evidence shows that silicone gel breast implants cause CTDs.

For More Information

Silicone Breast Implants: Has Science Been Ignored? is a concise pamphlet that describes the events of the silicone gel implant controversy and explains how lawsuits were successful despite medical evidence that silicone gel implants were safe. It is available through the American Council on Science and Health, 1995 Broadway, 2nd Floor, New York, NY, 10023-5860. Phone 212-362-7044.

Since the 1992 FDA ban, silicone gel has remained the implant of choice in Europe. (Interestingly, the FDA did not ban silicone gel testicular implants, even though they are identical in composition to silicone gel breast implants.)

Because silicone gel implants have never been shown to cause connective tissue disorders, plastic surgeons expect them to be back on the market in the United States sometime in the future. Because they provide a more natural look and feel than saline implants, plastic surgeons anticipate that they will once again be very popular. Until that time, silicone gel implants will be available only to those seeking breast reconstruction (but not augmentation) as a part of a national study evaluating a return to this alternative.

Using Your Flabby Tummy

It is true that plastic surgeons use abdominal skin and fat for breast reconstruction following surgical removal of the breast for cancer. This procedure is called a TRAM (an acronym for *transverse rectus abdominis myocutaneous*) flap. Unfortunately, your surgeon cannot simply cut out skin and fat from your abdomen, plunk it down on your breast, and expect it to survive. In order for surgeons to create a TRAM flap and enable it to survive, they must perform extensive surgery on your abdomen and sacrifice at least one of the two main abdominal muscles. (The muscles must be moved in order to provide circulation to the skin and fat that is transferred to your breast area.) Because the operation carries a higher risk of problems than breast implant placement and recovery takes longer, it can be justified following mastectomy but not for cosmetic breast augmentation.

Fat Injection

Many women request to have fat removed from one part of their body through liposuction and then reinjected into their breasts for augmentation. Although appealing in theory, fat injections into the breast have proved dangerous. Unfortunately, they attract calcium deposits that, on mammograms, look just like the calcium deposits due to cancer. Doctors cannot tell whether the calcium deposits are due to previous fat injections or a new cancer.

Let us assume that following your fat injection, new calcifications are seen each time you have a mammogram. Because you are concerned about breast cancer, you undergo a biopsy each time. But year after year, none of the biopsies show cancer.

Then what if someday you do develop breast cancer? Wouldn't you and your doctor be likely to assume that calcification on your mammogram was from fat? Wouldn't you be less likely to have another biopsy? Because the best chance for curing breast cancer is in its early stages, a delay in diagnosis could have fatal consequences.

In short, women who have fat injected into their breasts may face otherwise unnecessary breast biopsies and delay in diagnosis of true breast cancer, if it ever occurs. Then, too, injected fat sometimes fails to survive. If so, it may form hard lumps, cause pain, and distort the breast.

Although fat injection for breast augmentation has been condemned by plastic surgeons, it still is performed in the United States today. If any doctor recommends this, do not consent to it. Consider this a strong indication that the doctor is unethical or unqualified.

Oil-Filled Implants

Implants filled with vegetable oil, such as peanut oil and soybean oil, are under study. Oil-filled implants tend to provide a better look and feel than saline implants. Although currently used in Europe, the lengthy FDA approval process will delay their availability in the United States.

Breast Augmentation with Saline Implants: A Process of Making Choices

A number of important decisions precede your breast augmentation, such as implant position, size, shape, volume, and surface. The decisions you and your surgeon make before surgery will affect your risk of postoperative problems and your overall satisfaction. You will see that these decisions are complex: each option has pluses as well as minuses. You must decide which advantages are most important and which disadvantages you can accept. Effective communication between you and your surgeon is essential for the best outcome. If your surgeon does not involve you in these decisions, you may ask to be involved—or choose to see another surgeon.

As of this writing, saline implants are the only real option in the United States for cosmetic breast augmentation. If by the time you read this chapter, silicone gel implants have become available again, know that many of the issues explained here apply to silicone gel implants as well.

Risks of Breast Implants

As with all surgery, certain risks are inherent in breast augmentation (see Table 7-1). Read this section carefully, as the decisions you will make hinge on your understanding of the risks. An in-depth discussion with your plastic surgeon is also essential to understanding these potential problems.

Capsular Contracture

Scar tissue forms around all implanted materials as a natural part of healing. Scar tissue around a breast implant is not troublesome unless it tightens. An abnormally tight scar is known as a *capsular contracture*. It may develop months or years after implant placement. Plastic surgeons do not know why but have many theories.

The risk of developing a capsular contracture ranges from 10 to 50 percent, depending on which study is quoted. It appears that 50 percent of women with implants get at least mild capsular contractures and 10 percent get severe ones.

Capsular contractures, regardless of severity, do not need to be treated unless the woman who has them seeks improvement. Capsular contractures were previously treated by a procedure known as closed capsulotomy. Closed capsulotomy was a nonsurgical office procedure in which the surgeon manually squeezed the implanted breast, sometimes with tremendous force. This disrupted the surrounding scar, thereby softening the breast. Plastic surgeons now condemn this procedure because of its propensity to cause implant rupture, implant displacement, hematoma, unnatural appearance, and redevelopment of capsular contracture. If your surgeon suggests closed capsulotomy, you may wisely choose to seek another opinion.

When Can I Stop Worrying About Complications?

Most complications occur within a predictable time following surgery. If you do not develop them within the time periods noted, you can fairly conclude that you are probably free of these complications.

TIME SINCE SURGERY	POSSIBLE COMPLICATION
1 *day*	*Nipple numbness*
4 *weeks*	*Infection*
4 *weeks*	*Hematoma*

Capsular contracture, implant displacement, rippling, sloshing, and implant deflation may each occur at any time. Like any person who has synthetic implants, you can never conclude that you are free of complications.

Classification of Capsular Contractures

Mild: *The breast feels slightly firm, and the implant edges can be felt through the skin.*

Moderate: *The breast feels firm, and the implant can be both felt and perceived visually through the skin. The breast may appear unnaturally round or spherical.*

Severe: *The breast is hard, distorted, and painful.*

Table 7-1 *Risks of Breast Augmentation*
___

Capsular contracture

Interference with mammography

Implant displacement

*Implant deflation**

*Rippling**

*Sloshing**

Infection

Nipple Numbness

Hematoma
___

Saline implants only.

Current treatment involves surgical removal of the scar tissue and placement of a new implant. Recovery is similar to a first-time breast augmentation. If you have a moderate or severe capsular contracture, you may choose to undergo this operation. Realize, however, that capsular contracture may happen again; additional surgery is not guaranteed to solve your problem.

If your contracture is mild, as many are, you will likely chose to avoid surgery and simply live with it. Some plastic surgeons think implant exercises (explained later) may improve mild contractures.

Interference with Mammography

Breast augmentation does not increase the risk of breast cancer. Women who have breast implants may develop breast cancer, but their risk is the same as it is for women who do not have implants.

However, breast implants do interfere with the ability of a breast x-ray, or mammogram, to evaluate all breast tissue. (Because one in nine women in the United States will develop breast cancer in her lifetime, x-ray screening for early diagnosis is recommended.) The presence of a breast implant may, therefore, delay the diagnosis of breast cancer. Implant manufacturers, with the help of plastic surgeons, are trying to develop implants that do not obscure mammography. However, these will not likely become available for several years.

If you have a mother or sister with breast cancer, you are at increased risk for developing breast cancer. Because of the detection problem, you should carefully reconsider breast augmentation. If you insist on proceeding, ask your surgeon to place them under the muscle (explained later).

A special mammogram method is designed for women with breast implants. Called the Ecklund technique, all mammography facilities in the United States are required to offer it. (To obtain a list of mammography facilities in your state accredited by the American College of Radiology, call 800-227-6440.

Implant Displacement

Implants can displace from their original position. Capsular contracture may move an implant upward, inward, or outward, as shown in figure 7-1a–c. Or, a large-volume implant may drop, as shown in figure 7-1d. The larger the implant, the greater the likelihood of it dropping down. (To minimize this risk, choose a texture implant with a volume less than 350 ml and wear a support bra continuously for six weeks after surgery.) And the forces of healing may also move an implant out of position.

Interestingly, the nipple will point the direction opposite from where the implant has displaced. For example, if the implant moves upward, the nipple will appear to point downward (fig. 7-1a). Significant displacement will compromise the natural appearance of your breasts and will require an operation to re-center the implant.

Implant Deflation

Saline implants commonly develop a leak and deflate. Fortunately, implant deflation is not harmful, because the body simply absorbs the sterile saline. The deflated implant must be replaced with a new implant to reestablish breast symmetry.

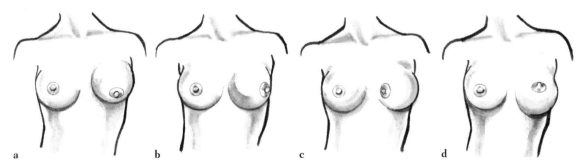

a   b   c   d

FIGURE 7–1: *Implant displacement. In each illustration, the implant on the left is in good position, while the implant on the right is displaced. Displacement shown is: (a) upward, (b) inward, (c) outward, and (d) downward ("dropped down"). In each case, the nipple appears to point in the direction opposite of implant displacement.*

The rate of deflation is about 1 to 4 percent per implant per year. In practical terms, if you have your implants for 25 years, there is a 25 to 100 percent chance that each one will deflate. Currently, manufacturers offer a lifetime warranty on their implants. If deflation occurs, they provide a new implant at no charge and pay up to $1,200 to defray the facility and anesthesia fees. They do not contribute anything toward the surgeon's fee.

Rippling

In a saline implant, the liquid moves freely within the implant and can cause small waves like those seen on the surface of a pond. These waves can be transmitted to the skin, causing the breast to wrinkle or ripple on its inner and lower sides. Rippling gives the breast an unnatural appearance. Thin women are particularly prone to rippling because they have less soft tissue covering their implants.

Rippling might be improved by replacing your implant or by putting more fluid in your existing implant, both of which require surgery. Rippling can sometimes be impossible to eliminate.

TRACY, a 34-year-old pharmaceutical representative, was relaxing in the tub one evening five years after breast augmentation. She became alarmed when she noticed that her right breast was shrinking by the minute. There was no obvious cause and no discomfort—simply a shrinking breast for no apparent reason. She was relieved to learn that this problem was not an emergency. One week later, her deflated right implant was replaced with a new one in the operating room. Although the prospect of surgery was less than appealing, the implant manufacturer provided a replacement implant and gave her money to help defray the hospital and anesthesia fees.

Sloshing

With saline implants, some women are troubled by a sloshing sensation as liquid moves within the implant. Sloshing is felt or heard but not seen. The woman herself may hear it whereas others do not. Sloshing often improves on its own. At any rate, most women get used to it.

Infection

Infection, which can occur after any operation, is devastating when it follows breast augmentation. It may require hospitalization, intravenous antibiotics, and removal of the implant. After removal, the incision may be left open to allow the infection to drain. Three to six months after the skin has healed, a new implant can be placed. During that time, your breast asymmetry will be awkward. Fortunately, the risk of infection is less than 1 percent.

Nipple Sensation and Erection

Loss of nipple sensation occurs in 15 percent of women who undergo breast augmentation. Numbness is often temporary but can be permanent.

ANNA, *a 26-year-old land surveyor, said before breast augmentation that loss of nipple sensation would not matter to her. Nipple sensation was maintained, and to her pleasant surprise, her nipple sensation became important for sexual gratification.*

Fortunately, heightened nipple sensation is actually more common than loss of sensation. Improved sensation is likely due to improved body image and increased sexual confidence.

Breast augmentation surgery does not affect nipple erection, which is preserved even if sensation is lost.

Breast-Feeding

Neither breast-feeding ability nor milk content is altered following breast augmentation. The greatest problem associated with pregnancy following breast augmentation is the appearance of the breast. (See "Postpartum Droop" later in this chapter.)

Hematoma

A hematoma is a blood collection that may accumulate next to the implant. Most hematomas appear within a few days of implant placement and usually require an additional operation for removal. It increases the likelihood of capsular contracture and of infection. The overall risk of hematoma is less than 2 percent, but it is higher in those who take aspirin or ibuprofen and in those who return to a physically demanding occupation or resume exercise shortly after surgery.

Decisions to Make Before Surgery

Prior to surgery, a number of decisions must be made, impacting your cosmetic result and your risk of complications. Reaching the best decisions can be challenging. Carefully consider each option by weighing its pluses and minuses (see Table 7-2). Prioritize your goals and base your choices on the issues that are most important to you. Communicate your goals to your surgeon, who will guide you through these decisions. The decisions include:

Implant position	*Above or below the muscle?*
Implant surface	*Smooth or textured?*
Implant shape	*Teardrop or round?*
Implant volume	*How big?*
Implant fill	*Fill to capacity or overfill?*
Site of incision	*Under the breast, around the nipple, or under the arm?*

TABLE 7-2 *Options for Breast Implant Selection and Placment*

PREOPERATIVE DECISION	ADVANTAGES	DISADVANTAGES
Implant position		
Above the muscle	• *Less discomfort* • *Less swelling* • *Faster recovery* • *No breast distortion when flexing pectoralis muscle*	• *Higher risk of capsular contractures* • *More interference with mammography* • *Worse cosmetic result in women with petite breasts*
Below the muscle	• *Lower risk of capsular contractures* • *Less interference with mammography* • *Better cosmetic result in women with petite breasts*	• *More discomfort* • *More swelling* • *Lengthier recovery* • *Possible breast movement with use of the pectoralis muscle*
Implant surface		
Smooth	• *Lower risk of rippling* • *Cost $100 less per pair than textured implants*	• *Higher risk of displacement*
Textured	• *Lower risk of displacement*	• *Higher risk of rippling* • *Costs $100 more per pair than smooth implants*
Implant shape		
Round	• *Rotation will not affect the appearance of breast* • *Cost is less than teardrop*	• *None*
Teardrop	• *May provide better cosmetic result in selected women according to some plastic surgeons*	• *May rotate, creating an abnormal shaped breast* • *Costs about $200 more than round implants*
Implant volume		
Less than 350 ml	• *Lower risk of displacement (dropping down)*	• *May be too small for women seeking large breast augmentation*
More than 400 ml	• *Adequate final size for women seeking large breast augmentation*	• *Higher risk of displacement*
Implant fill		
Fill to capacity	• *None*	• *Higher risk of deflation* • *Higher risk of rippling and sloshing*
Overfill	• *Lower risk of deflation* • *Lower risk of rippling and sloshing*	• *None*

TABLE 7-2 (*Continued*)

PREOPERATIVE DECISION	ADVANTAGES	DISADVANTAGES
Site of incision		
Under breast	• Scar heals inconspicuously and is hidden by the breast • Allows your plastic surgeon the best visibility during surgery	• If scar heals poorly, it may be visible when you are lying down unclothed
Around nipple	• Scar can be camouflaged around the nipple	• Because the scar is at the focal point of the breast, any imperfection will be highly visible • May alter nipple sensation
Underarm	• Well-hidden scar	• Requires endoscopic equipment • Least favorable visibility for your surgeon

Implant Position

Implants can be placed in one of two positions: just under the breast, or under the pectoralis muscle (the muscle under the breast). Either way, they are centered under each breast and nipple.

ABOVE THE MUSCLE

Position of the implant under the breast but above the pectoralis muscle is known as *subglandular placement* (fig. 7-2b) and offers several advantages. This is a smaller operation with less discomfort and faster recovery. Your breasts immediately appear attractive because swelling is minimal. In athletic, muscular women it confers less breast distortion—that is, a more natural

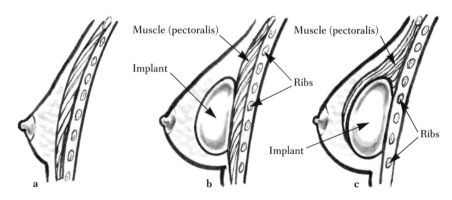

FIGURE 7–2: *Implant position. (a) A nonaugmented breast. (b) An implant above the muscle. (c) An implant below the muscle.*

result. It is also well suited to women who have adequate body fat or breast tissue to provide a cushion between the implant and the skin.

Disadvantages include a higher risk of capsular contracture and greater interference with mammography. Women with thin skin or petite breasts are likely to feel their implants through the skin.

BELOW THE MUSCLE

Implant position under the muscle (fig. 7-2c), also known as *submuscular* or *subpectoral placement,* offers the advantages of a lower rate of capsular contracture and less interference with mammography. Thin, nonathletic women with petite breasts may obtain their best cosmetic result with the implant placed under the muscle, which provides more padding between the implant and the skin.

Disadvantages begin with greater postoperative pain, greater swelling, and a longer recovery period. Pectoralis muscle swelling can be profound and may persist for weeks or months. During this time, the upper portion of the breast appears unnaturally full. And after swelling subsides, flexing the pectoralis muscles, such as during exercise, may cause the breasts to move and become distorted. Because athletic women will notice more breast distortion with activity, they should be deterred from submuscular placement.

Implant Surface

The outside surface of an implant can be either smooth or textured. The surface of the implant is indiscernible following surgery.

TEXTURED

Textured implants have a surface that feels like dull sandpaper. Once placed, textured implants tend to stay in position because the rough surface allows them to grip. They have been touted as bearing a lower risk of capsular contracture, although recent reports indicate that the rate of capsular contracture for smooth and textured implants may be comparable. The main disadvantage of textured implants is that they are more prone to rippling than smooth implants. They are also more prone to cause seromas, or fluid collections, around the implant. A minor disadvantage is that textured implants cost $100 more per pair than smooth. (Given the overall cost of breast augmentation surgery, this is not a significant amount.)

SMOOTH

Smooth implants offer the advantage of a lower rate of skin rippling, although they may have a higher rate of displacement when compared to textured implants. Following placement of smooth implants, you may be instructed to perform implant exercises (explained later).

Implant Shape

Implants may be teardrop-shaped or round. Round implants are shaped like a hamburger bun (fig. 7-3a). Teardrop implants are designed to have greater fullness toward the bottom (fig. 7-3b).

The selection of round versus teardrop implants is probably best left to your plastic surgeon, based on experience. Most plastic surgeons feel they can achieve comparably attractive and natural results with either shape. But because of fewer potential problems, 90 percent of surgeons recommend round implants.

TEARDROP

Because the breast has greater fullness toward the bottom, a few plastic surgeons prefer a teardrop implant, also called an anatomically shaped implant or an oval implant. They have found that teardrop implants provide a more natural result. Other surgeons think that the teardrop shape makes no difference, because as the body heals, it forces the implant into a round shape anyway.

Because of their design, teardrop implants must be oriented under the breast with the fullest portion at the bottom of the breast. One problem with teardrop implants is that they may rotate following surgery. This results in a sideways appearing breast. To reduce the risk of rotation, teardrop implants should be textured. Teardrop implants cost about $200 more than round implants. (This is an insignificant amount when considering the overall cost of this operation.)

ROUND

Round implants have several advantages. They may rotate freely under the breast without aesthetic consequences. They may be textured or smooth. Their cost is lower. Because the contents gravitate to the lower pole of the implant when a woman stands, the lower pole will naturally become full, thus negating the need for a teardrop implant.

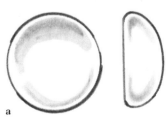
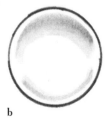
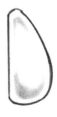

a   b

FIGURE 7–3: *Implant shape. (a) A round implant viewed from the front and side. (b) A teardrop implant viewed from the front and side.*

Implant Size

Deciding upon the right implant size is the hardest part of this operation. This is because cup size is not standardized. It varies between bra manufacturers and also among a single manufacturer's products. For example, the cup of a 32C bra is smaller than the cup of a 38C bra, even when made by the same company. So telling your surgeon which cup size you desire is of little help. Some surgeons may ask your desired cup size to get a general idea of your goals. Do not misinterpret this as a guarantee of final size.

Typically, implant sizes range from 6 to 18 fluid ounces, or 200–600 ml, although even larger and smaller implants are readily available. Implants are manufactured in 25-ml increments. As the volume of the implant grows, so does its diameter and projection.

Consider a number of factors when selecting an implant size.

• The larger the implant, the greater the potential for displacement. This can be a serious problem, so if you are seeking a large augmentation, be sure to discuss your concerns with your surgeon.

• It may be useful to discuss proportion with your surgeon. Many women seek augmentation to make their breasts proportionate to the rest of their bodies. Others may want their final size to be either larger or smaller than that. (Your surgeon may measure your breast diameter to select an implant size that will provide a proportionate augmentation.)

• Ask your surgeon to show you photographs of women with variably sized implants. Looking at photographs of other women whose preoperative breast size was similar to yours is most helpful. If you find an example of the size you desire, your surgeon can use the same size implant for you. If you feel the photographed breasts are either larger or smaller than the size you desire, this will also help your surgeon determine the best implant size for you.

• It is helpful to show your surgeon lingerie ads featuring women with breast sizes that are similar to your desired size.

• Ask your surgeon for breast implant samples or sizers. You can place these in your bra to help you determine the best volume. Or you may use water balloons that are filled to various volumes (a more arduous task). Some women find that purchasing a bra of their desired size makes either exercise easier.

• If you seek large breasts, do not hesitate to say so. The only way your surgeon can provide you with your desired result is if you are open about your goals. Now is not the time to be modest.

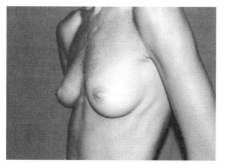 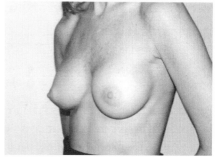

a   b

(a) Before breast augmentation. (b) After breast augmentation with 210 ml implants.

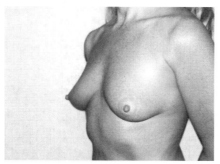 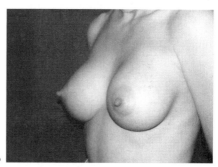

a   b

(a) Before breast augmentation. (b) After breast augmentation with 310 ml implants.

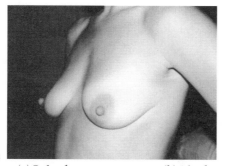 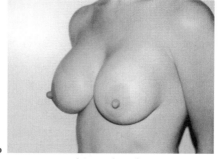

a   b

(a) Before breast augmentation. (b) After breast augmentation with 400 ml implants. The final size of the breasts appears similar to that of the woman who received 310 ml implants because they were initially smaller.

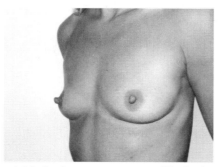

a   b

(a) Before breast augmentation. (b) After breast augmentation with 500 ml implants.

• Do not to tell your surgeon to simply place "average"-sized implants. The average size of implant placed in the United States in 1997 was 350 ml, whereas the average size of implant placed in 1998 was 450 ml. Either of these sizes may be too large or too small for some women, depending on their body size and their goals.

Communication is critical. The more honest you are with yourself and your plastic surgeon regarding your desired size, the more likely you will be pleased with your result. But remember, final breast size cannot be guaranteed.

Adjustable Implants

Because of the difficulty in determining the desired final breast size, some surgeons use adjustable saline implants. Adjustable implants have a small port that is placed under the skin in the underarm area. After surgery, your surgeon can easily and painlessly add or remove saline from your implant via this port, in the office. Clearly, adjustable implants allow you to have direct input regarding final volume.

The main drawback is that your desired size may still not be achieved. Your surgeon will have at most a 50 ml leeway in adjusting the volume. Adding or removing 50 ml does not alter breast size much. So you and your surgeon must still identify an implant size that is close to your desired size. A final disadvantage is that you will eventually require another operation to remove your ports. (This can usually be performed in the office under local anesthesia.) Because of these disadvantages, most surgeons do not use adjustable implants.

Implant Fill

Breast implants are empty when they arrive from the manufacturer. During surgery, surgeons fill each implant to the desired volume. They can adjust the amount within each implant before concluding the procedure.

Each implant holds a rated minimum volume, but it may be overfilled by 25–50 ml. Fill volume must be decided before or during surgery. Overfilling is commonly performed and reduces deflation, rippling, and sloshing. It is better to have a smaller implant overfilled than a larger implant filled to the rated capacity. (Implant manufacturers encourage overfilling and their warrantee currently covers overfilled implants.)

Deflation

Implants that are filled only to rated capacity (or less) tend to deflate. Their edges fold repeatedly and weaken, just as a piece of paper, folded along the same line repeatedly, thins and tears easily. That is why implant manufacturers recommend that implants be filled at least to the rated volume.

RIPPLING AND SLOSHING

If you have a waterbed, you may have noticed that the amount of water in the mattress alters its degree of rippling and sloshing. The same is true for saline breast implants. Both effects can be reduced by overfilling the implants.

OVER-OVERFILLING

Adding more saline beyond the usual overfilling point is also acceptable—and may in fact be desirable. For example, a "300-ml" implant may be overfilled to 350 ml, according to manufacturer specifications. Some surgeons will over-overfill the same implant to 400 or 450 ml, believing that this further reduces the risk of deflation, rippling, and sloshing. Over-overfilling does not necessarily void the manufacturer's warranty.

BREASTS OF DIFFERENT SIZES

If your breasts are different sizes, this can be addressed in one of three ways. Your surgeon will recommend the best option for you.

1. Have implants of different sizes placed. Because the implants will have different diameters, you may be introducing a new asymmetry. But, if your breasts vary significantly in size, this may be the best option.
2. Have identical implants placed and filled to different volumes. The less filled implant may slosh more, but this may only be temporary. This option may be most appropriate for mild to moderate asymmetry.
3. Have identical implants filled to the same volume. Your present size discrepancy will be less noticeable when both breasts are larger. This may be best for mild asymmetries.

Breast asymmetry is discussed again later in this chapter.

Site of Incision

Small incisions are possible even for a large implant, because an implant is not filled until it is in position. Incisions may be placed under the breast, around the nipple, under the arm, or in a preexisting scar (fig. 7-4).

UNDER THE BREAST

An incision under the breast, also called inframammary incision, is hidden along the natural skin crease, in the shadow of the breast. It heals inconspicuously and affords the surgeon excellent visibility for surgery. But if it heals poorly, it will be visible when you are lying down and wearing no clothing.

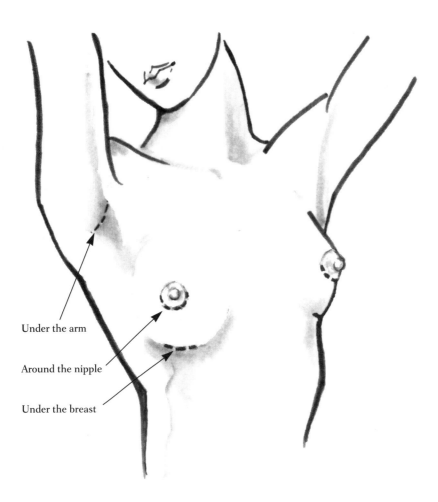

Under the arm

Around the nipple

Under the breast

FIGURE 7–4: *Incision options. The three common incisions used are under the arm, around the nipple, and under the breast. Each is shown with a dashed line. Only one incision is necessary for each breast.*

Around the Nipple

An incision around the nipple is designed to camouflage the scar by placing it at the junction of the nipple skin, called the areola, and the surrounding skin. Typically the incision goes halfway around the areola. Because of the natural color transition in this area, the scar is not easily seen. Many surgeons use this incision, also called the peri-areolar incision, with good results. However, because the nipple is the focal point of the breast, any imperfection, no matter how small, will be obvious. Also, there is a slightly higher risk of nipple numbness.

UNDER THE ARM

Using an endoscope (a pencil-sized rod with a fiber-optic camera on its tip), surgeons have achieved good cosmetic results with an incision under the arm, also called the transaxillary incision. Most surgeons use this technique only for smooth implants that are placed under the muscle. Placing textured implants above the muscle through this incision poses a greater technical challenge and therefore may not be offered.

The scar is well hidden. But if the scar remains noticeable after healing, it will be visible in evening gowns, tank tops, and bathing suits. It will be especially visible in women with olive or brown skin.

THROUGH THE BELLY BUTTON

Also called transumbilical breast augmentation, placement of implants can be performed through a small incision inside the belly button. This is mentioned only to be condemned. Use of this incision severely compromises your surgeon's view during the procedure, leading to an increased risk of intraoperative and postoperative complications. Implant manufacturers commonly void their warranty if the implants were placed through this incision.

THROUGH A PREVIOUS SCAR

A preexisting scar, such as a previous breast biopsy site, can be used if it is at least three centimeters (1¼ inches) long.

SCAR VISIBILITY

Usually scars from breast augmentation are hardly visible. Rarely do they become wide or unsightly. The final visibility of your scar depends more on your healing process than on your plastic surgeon's technique.

Aesthetic Issues

Breast Asymmetry

All women have breast asymmetry. One breast may be larger than the other. One breast may be shaped differently than the other. One breast may be higher or broader than the other. The nipples may be uneven in size, shape, position, or height. Your surgeon will probably point these asymmetries out to you prior to surgery. It is important that you recognize them and understand that, with the exception of breast size discrepancy, asymmetry will not be improved or corrected as a result of breast augmentation. In fact, some asymmetries may become more obvious. (Breast size discrepancy is addressed in "Implant Fill.")

Cleavage

Cleavage refers to the distance between the breasts, not to breast size. By way of cultural values, when the breasts are close together, they are considered to have attractive cleavage. For this reason, many women hope to gain cleavage as a result of their surgery. However, just because breasts are larger does not mean they will be closer together. In fact, breast augmentation does not change breast position or cleavage. If your breasts are widely spaced prior to surgery, they will remain widely spaced afterward.

Breast Droop

Droopy breasts may be improved through a breast lift operation (see Chapter 8). Expecting breast augmentation alone to solve this problem is usually a mistake. Some cases of mild droop may be improved through implant placement. However, improvement may be only temporary.

Stretch Marks

Breast augmentation will not improve stretch marks on the breasts. It may even make them worse or more obvious.

Breast Shape

Breast augmentation mainly affects breast volume, not shape. Some breast shapes are not amenable to simple augmentation. One example of this is a tubular breast, which is narrow and long. If your plastic surgeon tells you your breast is tubular, expect that more surgery will be necessary than just placement of implants.

What to Expect

Breast augmentation is an outpatient procedure. Discomfort is variable and will be controlled with prescription pain medication. You will be able to return to work within a week and may resume exercise within two to four weeks. Your final result will be evident within one to four months.

To help you to plan for and recover from your procedure, reread Steps 7 and 10 of Chapter 1.

Implant Exercises

Implant exercises are controversial among surgeons. Some think they are of value, others disagree.

If you have smooth implants, your surgeon may instruct you to start implant exercises one to two weeks following surgery and to perform them

Vital Statistics

Anesthesia: Sedation or general.

Location of operation: Office or hospital.

Length of surgery: 1–2 hours.

Length of stay: Outpatient (home same day).

Discomfort: Mild to moderate following implant placement over the muscle, and moderate to severe following implant placement under the muscle. Anticipate 3–14 days of pain medication. Ask your surgeon to inject long-lasting local anesthetic during surgery to make your first night more comfortable. Muscle relaxants also help, especially with submuscular implants.

Swelling: Improves in 3–10 days if the implant was placed above the muscle and 2–12 weeks if the implant was placed under the muscle. Swelling may be worse if you are athletic or if you resume upper body exercise within 2 weeks of surgery.

Bruising: Improves in 0–10 days. Some have no bruising.

Numbness: Temporary numbness, if it occurs, lasts 1–2 months. Permanent numbness occurs in 15 percent.

Bandages: Removed in 2–7 days.

Stitches: Most plastic surgeons use absorbable stitches that are buried under the skin and never require removal. If your surgeon uses nonabsorbable stitches, they will be visible outside the skin and will be removed in 5–7 days.

Support: You will wear a sports bra or Ace wrap for 1–4 weeks. Avoid an underwire bra until your surgeon approves it.

Work: You may return to work in 3–7 days if the implants were placed over your muscle, and 5–10 days if the implants were placed under your muscle. If your job requires lifting, wait 3–4 weeks.

Resume exercise: May be resumed in 2–4 weeks.

Final result: Will be seen within 1 month if the implants were placed under the breast and within 4 months if the implants were placed under the muscle.

once or twice daily (fig. 7-5). You will move your implants in all directions to stretch the scar around your implants and hopefully prevent capsular contractures. Because capsular contractures may occur months or years following implant placement, plan to continue implant exercises for as long as you have implants. Since scheduling time out of your day for this is a nuisance, you may simply plan to perform your implant exercises in the shower each morning.

If your implants are textured, avoid implant exercises. A presumed advantage of the rough texture is that it allows surrounding tissue to stick to the implant, so as to prevent displacement. Performing implant exercises might negate this benefit by freeing the implant from surrounding soft tissue.

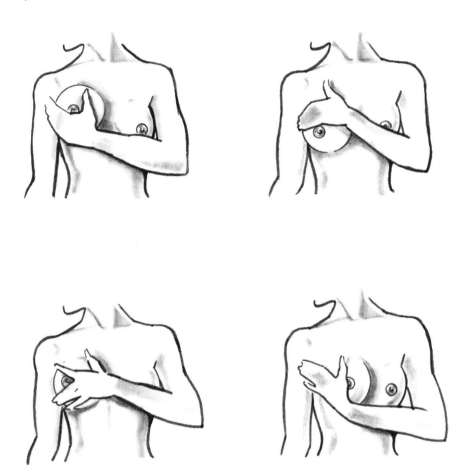

Figure 7–5: *Implant exercises. Women with smooth implants may be instructed to gently but firmly press on each implant in all directions once a day. These exercises may reduce the risk of capsular contracture.*

Adjusting to Your "New" Breasts

Getting used to your new breast size may be easy or difficult. Some women are immediately pleased with their size. Others may take months to adjust.

This type of roller coaster response to breast augmentation is not uncommon. It seems particularly more common in women with analytical minds.

Your new breasts will have more form and firmness than before surgery. They will feel less fleshy and slightly more stiff. When your body is exposed to cold temperatures, such as during swimming or snow skiing, saline implants may drop in temperature and may temporarily create a cool sensation in your chest.

Telltale Signs

Spherical Breast

Moderate or severe capsular contractures can cause the breasts to appear unnaturally round. Severely affected breasts can resemble coconuts. If you peruse *Sports Illustrated*'s swimsuit edition, you will see a variety of examples. (See the section on capsular contracture for treatment of this problem.)

Postpartum Droop

During pregnancy, breast skin stretches to accommodate the enlarging breast. Following pregnancy, the breast returns to normal size. The skin may not regain its tone and may allow the breast to droop. Because the implant does not droop, the breast may appear to have fallen off the implant (fig. 7-6). A breast lift operation is required to restore the breast to its natural position.

Not all women who become pregnant following augmentation suffer this cosmetic problem. Those who have minimal change in breast size during pregnancy and those with good skin tone are less likely to have postpartum droop.

JANET, *a 28-year-old mechanical illustrator, spent a great deal of time selecting the appropriately sized implant. Yet immediately following surgery, she felt that her breasts were far too large and that a mistake had been made. She was assured that the agreed upon implant size had been used, that her swelling accounted for some of her volume, and that most of her reaction was due to the sudden dramatic change in size for which no one can truly be prepared. She reluctantly agreed to let time pass before making her final judgment. Four weeks later, she said that she had become accustomed to them, but that they actually seemed too small. She was again convinced to wait. Two months later, she was finally satisfied with the size she chose.*

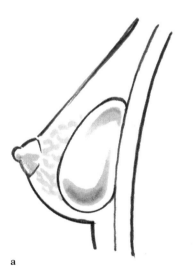 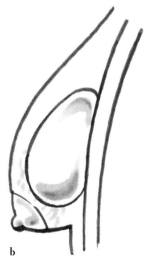

a   b

FIGURE 7–6: *Postpartum drop. (a) An augmented breast prior to pregnancy. (b) Following pregnancy, the breast droops, but the implant holds position. This creates the appearance of the breast falling off the implant.*

Symmastia

Symmastia is the merging of the breasts into an indistinct mass (fig. 7-7). It occurs if the skin between the breasts loses its attachment to the breast bone during surgery. This is a challenging problem to fix, and revision surgery may not be successful. Fortunately, symmastia is rare, with fewer than 1 percent of implant recipients developing it.

Cost

In the United States, the range of total fees for breast augmentation extends from $5,000 to $7,000. The average cost is:

Surgeon's fee	$ 3,100
Anesthesiologist's fee	$ 700
Operating room (facility) fee	$ 900
Implant fee	$ 1,300
Total	$6,000

See "Fees" in Chapter 1 for various factors that might affect your own actual cost.

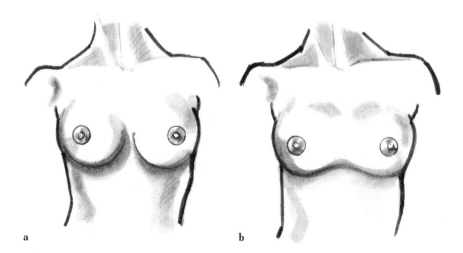

a   b

FIGURE 7–7: *Telltale sign, symmastia. (a) Natural breasts, which are distinct and separate. (b) Breasts with symmastia, which are unnaturally merged together into an indistinct mass.*

Implants cost $950 to $1,100 per pair from the manufacturer. Your surgeon or the operating facility will mark up that price to cover the cost of ordering, shipping, and stocking them. If you are charged more than $1,300 for your implants, you should question the price. Unfortunately, only plastic surgeons and hospitals may purchase implants, so you will be limited in your ability to negotiate.

Duration of Results

Breast implants are permanent and will not be absorbed or biodegraded by your body. They will remain in place unless you choose to have them removed. But they do sometimes deflate or cause other problems that significantly alter the result. (See "Risks of Breast Implants" for details.) If you have no such problems, your results should be lasting.

Need for Future Breast Operations

Breast implants may be associated with numerous problems, many of which require an operation for correction. These include:

Capsular contracture	*Hematoma*
Rippling	*Asymmetry*
Deflation	*Breast droop*
Infection	*Symmastia*
Displacement	

Not all women with implants require further breast surgery, but it is prudent to *assume that you will*. And anticipate lifelong annual follow-up visits with your plastic surgeon.

Another relatively common reason women seek additional surgery is to downsize their implants. With time, large implants may become physically burdensome. As young adults, women often request much larger implants than they desire decades later.

Changing Your Mind

Breast implants can be removed at any time. However, you may find your natural breasts have changed due to breast shrinkage and skin stretch.

Breast shrinkage, or atrophy, occurs to varying degrees in response to pressure exerted on your breast by the implant. Do not expect this to improve following implant removal.

After breast augmentation, your skin stretches to accommodate the new breast size. Following removal of the implant, your skin may tighten—but it may not regain its original tone. Your breasts may droop. The greater your skin laxity, the greater your droop. In severe cases, your breasts may resemble empty socks. (Breasts may also droop as a result of normal aging.)

The degree of skin tightening following implant removal depends on your age, the length of time the implant was in place, and the volume of the implant. An older woman with large implants placed decades earlier should expect little tightening of breast skin and greater droop. A younger woman with smaller implants can expect more tightening and less droop. If tightening does not occur to a satisfactory degree within six months, breast lift is an option (see Chapter 8).

ANDREA, *an uninhibited 33-year-old computer salesperson, was so pleased with her implants that after a few drinks at a large family picnic, she proudly pulled open her shirt to show off her new breasts. Subsequently two family members sought breast augmentation.*

Satisfaction

Breast augmentation is one of the most requested procedures in plastic surgery. As with all cosmetic surgery, there are no guarantees regarding outcome or satisfaction. If you understand and accept the risks of this operation and still choose to proceed, you most likely will be glad you did.

Concluding Thoughts

The decision to proceed with breast augmentation is not a simple one, particularly in light of the fact that those who receive implants should anticipate future revision. Although breast implants do not cause medical illnesses, there are numerous risks associated with their placement. Those who understand these issues and choose to proceed with breast augmentation are among the most satisfied patients in any plastic surgery practice.

Questions to Ask Your Plastic Surgeon

Will the implants be placed above or below the muscle?

Will the implants be smooth or textured? Round or teardrop?

Where will the incisions be?

Do you plan to overfill the implants?

May I see before-and-after pictures of women with variously sized implants?

Will you use long-lasting local anesthetic at the time of surgery?

May I have muscle relaxants after surgery?

What is your policy regarding revision surgery?

Tips and Traps

Thin and small-breasted women should favor implant placement under the muscle. The advantages of less interference with mammography, less rippling, and more cushion between the implant and the skin outweigh the drawbacks, many of which are temporary.

Athletic women should favor placement of the implant above the muscle to avoid breast distortion when the pectoral muscles are flexed.

Round implants are appropriate for most women. Compared to teardrop implants, they provide an aesthetically similar result, do not restrict options regarding implant surface, obviate the potential problem of implant rotation, and cost less.

Request overfilling of your implants to reduce the risk of deflation, rippling, and sloshing.

Do not expect tight cleavage if your breasts are widely separated now. Implants do not change the position of your breasts—only the volume.

Anticipate that your breasts will look and feel more stiff than is natural. If this is not acceptable, wait for other implant options to become available.

Avoid exercise for 3–4 weeks to minimize swelling and the risk of seroma and hematoma.

Women whose mother or sister had breast cancer should recognize that they are at increased risk for breast cancer and that implants may delay their diagnosis.

Women unwilling to accept the potential loss of nipple sensation should not have breast augmentation.

Women unwilling to accept the potential need for further surgery should not have breast augmentation.

Women planning to have children should consider deferring breast augmentation.

Since lifelong follow-up is important, find out if your surgeon charges for visits after surgery. Many do not.

8

Enhancing Droopy Breasts

Breast Lift

*B*reast lift is an entirely different operation than breast augmentation. *Breast lift* (also called *mastopexy*) affects the position of the breasts without affecting size. It is primarily for women who have droopy breasts and who would like the same-sized breasts to be restored to a more youthful position. *Augmentation* affects size, and usually does not affect position. It is for women who wish to have larger breasts (see Chapter 7).

Causes of Breast Droop

Breast droop is an unfortunate by-product of breast size, age, gravity, and pregnancy. Each of these causes contributes to loosening or stretching of the breast skin. Because breast skin is solely responsible for holding the breast in position, its laxity will give way to breast droop, also called breast *ptosis* (pronounced "toe-sis").

If your breast skin is tight and has good tone, it will hold your breast high. If your skin is loose or stretched, it will allow your breast to droop.

Size, Age, and Gravity

Breast size is the greatest determinant of droop. As breasts enlarge, they are pulled downward by gravity. The overlying skin stretches and loses its tone.

> **JOYCE** *felt much older than her 44 years because of breasts that sagged halfway to her belly button. She was satisfied with her breast size, but frustrated by the effects of gravity. Following breast lift, her breast size remained the same, and her breasts were restored to a higher and more youthful position.*

Age also contributes to breast droop, because the skin thins with age and becomes less resistant to the effects of gravity.

Size is a more important factor than age. A 20-year-old woman with large breasts will have greater droop than a 50-year-old woman with small breasts. Age, however, does play a role, because breasts will droop progressively over time, regardless of their size.

Pregnancy

During pregnancy, your breasts enlarge, causing the skin to stretch. Following pregnancy your breasts diminish in size, but the overlying skin may not. It often loses tone and allows droop. You should defer breast lift until after your last child is born; otherwise future pregnancy will cause droop to recur.

Degrees of Breast Droop

Plastic surgeons gauge droop based on the position of the nipple compared to the breast crease, also called the *inframammary crease* (fig. 8-1). The ideal position for the nipple is above the inframammary crease, but with time, age and gravity, the breast descends.

How Breast Lift Works

As the cause of breast droop is loose skin, the treatment is to remove excess skin. The remaining, tighter skin then holds the breast in a higher position. The greater the droop, the more skin must be removed—and the more exten-

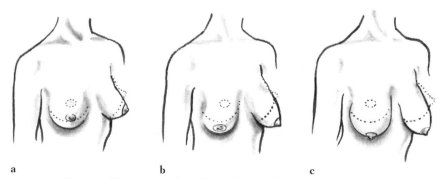

a   b   c

FIGURE 8-1: *Degrees of breast droop. Dotted lines show ideal breast position. (a) Mild droop; the nipple is level with the inframammary crease. (b) Moderate droop; the nipple is below the inframammary crease. (c) Advanced droop; the nipple is on the lowest part of the breast, pointing downward.*

sive will be the scars. The operation reduces nipple size to 1½ inches in diameter, an aesthetic and appropriate size for most women.

Breast lift involves trading one cosmetic problem for another, as droop is improved at the cost of new scars. Therefore, many women are unwilling to consider this operation unless their droop is advanced.

The following are general guidelines. Ask your plastic surgeon which procedure is most appropriate in your case.

Mild Droop

Correction of mild droop usually involves removal of skin around the nipple, which leaves a relatively well-hidden scar (fig. 8-2).

Moderate Droop

Surgeons usually correct moderate droop by removing skin both around and below the nipple, resulting in scars in both areas (fig. 8-3).

Advanced droop

Correction of advanced droop usually involves skin removal and scars in three areas: around the nipple, below the nipple, and along the inframammary crease (fig. 8-4).

Purse-String Breast Lift

Another alternative is a purse-string mastopexy, in which a donut of skin is removed from around the nipple, regardless of the extent of droop. This limits

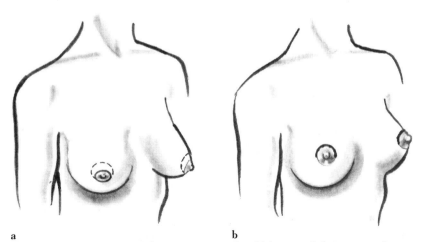

a   b

FIGURE 8-2: *Breast lift for mild droop. (a) Breasts with mild droop, with the anticipated incision (dashed line). (b) Following surgery, the breast is lifted and the scar is above the nipple (solid line). For correction of mild droop, the scar often extends all the way around the nipple.*

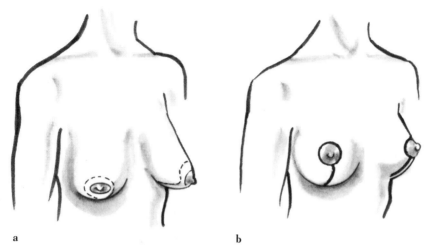

a   b

FIGURE 8-3: *Breast lift for moderate droop. (a) Breasts with moderate droop, with the anticipated incision (dashed line). (b) Following surgery, the breasts are lifted and the scar is present around the nipple and from the nipple to the inframmary crease (solid line).*

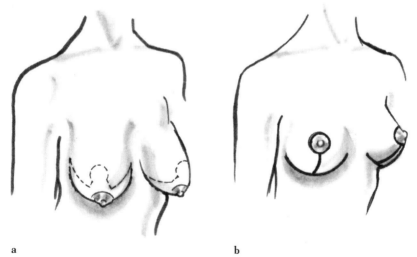

a   b

FIGURE 8-4: *Breast lift for advanced droop. (a) Breasts with advanced droop, with the anticipated incision (dashed line). (b) Following surgery, the breasts are lifted and the scar is more
extensive (solid line).*

the scar to the area around the nipple, but there may be drawbacks such as flattening of the breasts, widening of the areola, which is the pigmented skin
around the nipple, and development of stretch marks.

Breast Augmentation to Improve Breast Droop

Breast Augmentation and Lift

Breast implants will slightly improve breast position. If your droop is mild, then it is possible that augmentation alone may remedy this problem. However, it will not raise moderately droopy breasts. Also, the lift you get from augmentation may be only temporary. If you have droopy breasts and desire improvement, a breast lift may be the most reliable option.

Women who desire both larger and higher breasts may seek to combine breast augmentation and lift. Many plastic surgeons perform both procedures concurrently. Others recommend that the lift and augmentation be performed separately for the best cosmetic outcome. Your surgeon will definitely have an opinion on this matter.

Incisions and Scars

Breast lift is designed to keep all scars at or below the nipple level. They will not be visible in clothing or most swimwear. Immediately following surgery, the scars may be red, firm, and raised. The scars will mature, fade, and soften within 3 to 12 months. Many scars fade and become nearly invisible, but other scars may become wide and raised. Final scar appearance cannot be predicted prior to surgery.

Scars are permanent. Not all women consider the scars to be acceptable, even when well healed and barely visible. Many women who initially seek breast lift surgery reconsider after learning about the scars. Women who accept the exchange of droop for scars tend to be satisfied with the result, as long as they understand that scars are permanent.

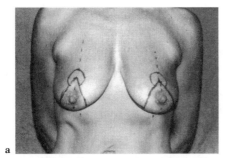 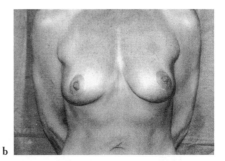

(a) Moderate breast droop, before breast lift. Circles indicate the anticipated position of the nipples. (b) After breast lift.

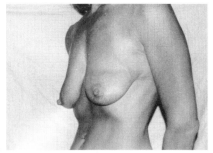 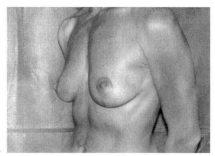

(a) Moderate breast droop, before breast lift. (b) After breast lift.

What to Expect

Breast lifts are most commonly performed under sedation or general anesthesia. You will be allowed to go home the same day. Discomfort is mild to moderate and will be controlled with prescription pain medication. You will be able to return to work within a week. Your final result will be evident after your scars have matured, which takes about six months.

To help you to plan for and recover from your procedure, reread Steps 7 and 10 of Chapter 1.

Vital Statistics

Anesthesia: General or sedation.

Location of operation: Office or hospital.

Length of surgery: 1–2 hours (3–4 hours if performed with augmentation).

Length of stay: Outpatient (home same day).

Discomfort: Mild to moderate. Anticipate 2–7 days of prescription pain medication.

Swelling and bruising: Improve in 3–10 days.

Bandages: Will be removed in 1–7 days.

Stitches: Most plastic surgeons use absorbable stitches that are buried under the skin and never require removal. Nonabsorbable stitches will be visible outside the skin and will be removed in 5–7 days.

Support: Wear a sports bra or Ace wrap for 1–4 weeks. Avoid an underwire bra until your surgeon approves it.

Back to work: You may return to work in 3–7 days.

Exercise: May be resumed in 2 weeks.

Final result: Will be seen after the scars have matured, which will be about 6 months.

Complications

When your operation is performed by a qualified plastic surgeon, both your procedure and recovery will likely be uneventful. Even in ideal circumstances, however, complications may occur. In addition to the specific complications mentioned here, refer to Chapter 1 for general complications that may follow any procedure.

Skin Death

Skin may die if it is closed under excessive tension, or if you smoke. If skin death occurs, you will develop an open wound, usually in a small area below the nipple. The wound will heal within weeks, depending on its size. Final appearance cannot be predicted; some open wounds actually heal more discreetly than do scars.

Nipple Problems

Loss of nipple sensation, change of nipple color, and partial nipple death may occur. The likelihood is greatest among those with severely droopy breasts, but remains rare. If numbness occurs, nipple sensation usually returns within six months. Color changes and irregularities may never improve.

When Can I Stop Worrying About Complications?

Most complications occur within a predictable time following surgery. If you do not develop them within the time period noted, you can fairly conclude that you are probably free of these complications:

Time After Surgery	Possible Complication
3 days	*Loss of nipple sensation*
2 weeks	*Partial nipple death*
1 month	*Change in nipple color*

Telltale Signs

The main telltale signs of breast lift are scars, which have been fully discussed throughout this chapter.

High Nipple

If your nipple is too high after surgery, it will look unnatural (fig. 8-5). It will likely worsen over time because your breast mound will descend in response to gravity, but your nipple will not. Attempts to correct this problem can result in new scars that will be visible in bathing suits and low-cut clothing.

Reasons Not to Have a Breast Lift

To avoid the need for repeat breast lift, those planning to have children should wait until after the last child is born.

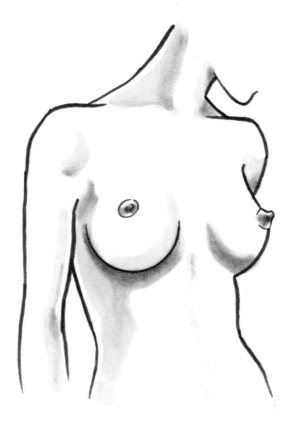

FIGURE 8-5: *Both nipples are high and appear to point upward. If your nipple is placed too high, you may have this undesirable telltale result.*

Smokers who are unable to quit smoking at least two weeks before surgery should defer surgery.

Cost

In the United States, the range of total fees for breast lift extends from $4,000 to $7,000. The average cost is:

Surgeon's fee	$3,400
Anesthesiologist's fee	$ 800
Operating room (facility) fee	$ 1,100
Total	$5,300

With breast augmentation at the same time, the national average is $9,500. For both procedures in New York, expect to pay an average of $15,000.

See "Fees" in Chapter 1 for various factors that might affect your own actual cost.

Duration of Results

Due to ongoing aging and gravity, the long-term result of a breast lift is difficult to predict. The larger your breasts, the sooner and greater they will re-droop. Lifts on small breasts may last indefinitely; those on large breasts may last just months. If droop recurs, additional lifts can be performed.

Satisfaction

Breast lift exchanges the aesthetic problem of droop for the aesthetic problem of scars. Those who have a clear understanding of this drawback and choose to proceed with surgery are usually satisfied with their results. Disappointment may be due to complications, misconceptions about scars, or recurrence of droop.

Questions to Ask Your Plastic Surgeon

Will a breast implant alone solve the problem of my droopy breasts?

Will you show me where the scars will be on my breasts?

How long will a breast lift last in my case?

Concluding Thoughts

Breast lift offers you the opportunity for youthful breast position, without affecting size. If you desire larger breasts, breast lift can be performed together with augmentation. The main drawback of breast lift is scarring. Because scars represent a different cosmetic problem than droop, each woman must decide if this trade-off is worthwhile.

Tips and Traps

Anticipate scars. As a general rule, the more extensive your droop, the more extensive will be your scars.

Scars can be limited to the area around the nipple if droop is mild. If droop is moderate or advanced, limiting your scars to this area may impose further trade-offs such as flattening of the breast and stretch marks.

Wait until you are done bearing children before considering breast lift.

Quit smoking for at least two weeks before surgery.

Anticipate recurrent droop if your breasts are large. The larger your breasts are, the more droop you can expect, and the sooner you can expect it.

9

Tightening Your Tummy and Bringing Up the Rear

Tummy Tuck, Thigh Lift, and Body Lift

As you age, you begin to see the effects of time and gravity on your abdomen, thighs, and buttocks. Compound this with the consequences of pregnancy, and the result is a flabby abdomen, sagging thighs, and droopy buttocks. Even rigid diets and vigorous exercise will not tighten loose skin or raise fallen parts.

Fortunately, cosmetic surgery has something to offer. If your problem is a protuberant abdomen with loose skin, a tummy tuck may be appropriate. For loose inner thigh skin, an inner thigh lift may be the operation of choice. If your buttocks and outer thighs have descended, lifting these areas can help. Those with concerns in all areas may consider a total body lift, which combines tummy tuck, inner thigh lift, and outer thigh/buttock lift.

Following a tummy tuck, thigh lift, buttock lift, or body lift, you will find that your skin is tighter and your body leaner. (In contrast, liposuction plays only a minor role in skin tightening. Generally, liposuction will make your body appear thinner, whereas a body lift will make it look younger.)

These operations, however, are not appropriate for all women. Each procedure represents major surgery, poses significant risks, and is worthy of serious deliberation. To determine if they are right for you, consult a plastic surgeon who is experienced in body contour surgery.

BOBBIE, *a 58-year-old owner of a small shop, underwent a face-lift, eyelid surgery, and forehead lift. She felt 10 years younger when she looked in the mirror. When she looked lower, however, she felt old and droopy again. After four pregnancies, her abdomen bulged and her buttocks drooped. A total body lift brought her body into harmony with her new face.*

Tummy Tuck

Tummy tuck, also called "abdominoplasty," is an operation primarily for women who have been pregnant. Pregnancy stretches the abdominal wall and can result in a flabby and protuberant abdomen.

The term "tummy tuck" is deceptive and implies a simple, risk-free operation. In truth, tummy tuck is neither simple nor risk-free. It is a serious operation with potentially serious consequences. If a surgeon tells you that tummy tuck is minor surgery, go elsewhere.

ANGIE, a 39-year-old mother of three, was often asked her due date. Although she had a protuberant abdomen, she certainly was not pregnant. Because of her previous pregnancies, she had loose skin and a lax inner girdle (see below). After a tummy tuck, she could fit into clothing four sizes smaller and, as she put it, no longer looked as though she was "a member of the stork club."

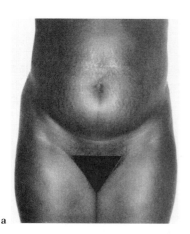

a

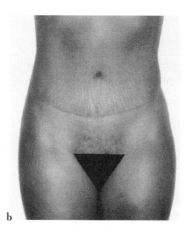

b

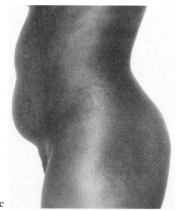

c

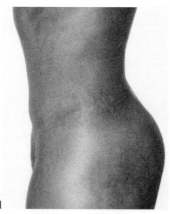

d

(a and c) Before tummy tuck.   *(b and d) After tummy tuck.*

Tummy Tuck or Liposuction

CINDY, a 39-year-old freelance photographer, requested liposuction of her abdomen. On examination, however, she had excess fat, a lax inner girdle, loose skin, and was better suited to a tummy tuck. She was insistent on liposuction because she thought tummy tucks were too extensive and the scar too long. She sought liposuction from another surgeon, and not surprisingly continued to have a bulging abdomen and loose skin. She finally had a tummy tuck and has been satisfied since. In looking back, she regrets that she had not listened to the original advice.

Women often question whether their lax abdomens would be best improved by tummy tuck or liposuction. The answer depends on whether your problem is due to loose skin, excess fat, lax inner girdle, or a combination of these. In order to determine your problems, work through the "Abdominal Self-Assessment" sidebar.

Tummy Tuck Versus Liposuction

Tummy tuck can improve loose skin, excess fat, and lax fascia. Liposuction will only reduce excess fat. It will not improve a lax inner girdle, nor will it significantly tighten loose skin.

If you have excess fat, tight skin, and tight abdominal fascia, you will be a candidate for abdominal liposuction. If you have excess skin, poor skin tone, or lax fascia, then you will be disappointed with the results of liposuction. A tummy tuck will be more appropriate.

Stretch marks are an indication of poor skin tone. If you have abdominal stretch marks, you will be far better suited to a tummy tuck.

Abdominal Self-Assessment

Stand in front of your mirror and evaluate your bare abdomen. Do not tighten your muscles. Relax. You will be assessing three characteristics: skin, fat, and inner girdle.

Skin

Pinch the skin of your lower abdomen. See if you can get the skin near your belly button to meet the skin near your pubic hair. If so, you have significantly loose skin.

Fat

Tighten your abdominal muscles by trying to flatten your tummy. With your abdomen tight, pinch your skin and fat. If you can gather more than a fistful, you probably have excess fat. Tightening your abdomen helps you to distinguish between excess fat and a loose inner girdle.

Inner Girdle

Both your inner girdle and your abdominal muscles, the rectus muscles, affect the tone and appearance of your abdomen. Your inner girdle is made of fascia. If you are a meat eater, you have seen fascia, which is the dense white tissue that surrounds steak ("gristle"). A broad sheet of fascia extends from your rib cage to your pubic bone. The purpose of fascia is to keep abdominal contents, such as stomach and intestines, inside the abdomen. (In this chapter, the terms "abdominal fascia" and "inner girdle" are used interchangeably.)

During pregnancy, your inner girdle stretches to accommodate the growing fetus. Following pregnancy, your inner girdle may or may not regain the tone it once had, depending on how distended your abdomen became, how old you were during pregnancy, and how many pregnancies you have had. (Younger mothers have a better opportunity to regain fascia tone. For some, improving muscle tone through exercise will solve this problem.)

Stand with your profile toward the mirror and tighten your abdomen. You will see the effects of muscle tone on the appearance of your abdomen. When your abdominal muscles relax, the appearance of your abdomen is determined mostly by your inner girdle (fig. 9-1). The visible difference between a relaxed abdomen and a tightened abdomen reflects the degree of weakness in your abdominal fascia. If there is a significant difference, you likely have significant laxity of your fascia. This is a critical point to assess. If you have a lax inner girdle, tightening it through tummy tuck is one of the keys to a more aesthetic abdomen.

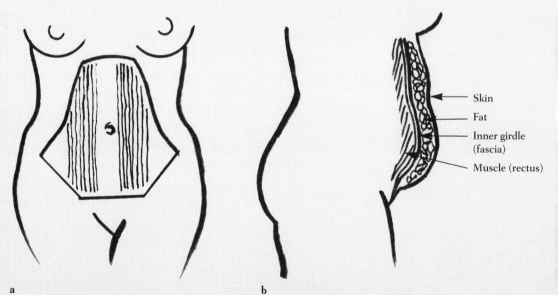

a   b

FIGURE 9-1: *Abdominal self-assessment for skin, fat, and fascia. (a) A frontal view showing the inner girdle beneath the skin. The verticle lines indicate the position of the paired rectus muscles under the inner girdle. (b) A side view, showing that a bowed inner girdle can cause the skin and fat to bow forward also.*

JULIA, *a 35-year-old mother of three, wanted to regain the taut, flat abdomen of her youth. Following her pregnancies, she had developed loose skin, lax inner girdle, and significant excess abdominal fat. It was evident that liposuction alone would not be adequate, because it would not improve her lax fascia and loose skin. Tummy tuck alone would not be adequate, because it would not address the problem of excess upper abdominal fat. In order to achieve the desired results safely, she underwent tummy tuck followed by liposuction four months later. Although she would have preferred to have both procedures simultaneously, she was grateful for an uncomplicated recovery and a satisfactory final result.*

ANNA, *a 43-year-old data processor, sought laser removal of stretch marks on her lower abdomen. She was surprised and disappointed to learn that lasers were not successful in removing stretch marks (see Chapter 13). During her consultation, she also complained about her protrusive abdomen. After examination, it was apparent that a tummy tuck would improve both problems. Tummy tuck removed all excess skin below her belly button, both removing her stretch marks and flattening her abdomen.*

Tummy Tuck and Liposuction

Tummy tuck removes fat of the lower abdomen only. If you have significant excess upper abdominal fat as well as lax fascia and loose skin, you may need both tummy tuck and liposuction. However, performing abdominal liposuction and tummy tuck simultaneously increases the risk of serious complications such as skin death. For this reason, many surgeons will not perform both at the same time and recommend separating the operations by at least three months.

Some surgeons will perform limited liposuction of the abdomen at the same time as tummy tuck, but most will avoid extensive abdominal liposuction. Concurrent liposuction of non-abdominal areas such as the hips or thighs does not increase the risk of abdominal skin complications.

Stretch Marks

Lower abdominal stretch marks are removed during tummy tuck. Fortunately, most stretch marks occur on the lower abdomen.

Stretch marks at the level of your belly button may or may not be removed with a tummy tuck. Stretch marks above your belly button will not be removed.

Hips

Standing in front of a mirror, look at your hips objectively. Does your silhouette follow a single gentle curve from your waist, around your hips, and down your thigh? Or does your silhouette more closely resemble a cello? If so, your hips form a bulge and your outer thighs form a bulge, much like the silhouette of a cello (fig. 9-2).

A tummy tuck may narrow your waist, because it will tighten your fascia horizontally (fig. 9-3). However, it will not narrow your hips. As a result, your hips may appear larger in comparison to your tightened waist. Your plastic surgeon may recommend liposuction of your hips in addition to tummy tuck.

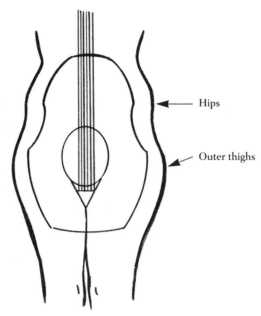

FIGURE 9-2: *The cello silhouette. If you have this type of silhouette, your hips will form the upper bulge, and your outer thighs the lower bulge.*

Do not be offended and do not assume your plastic surgeon is pitching unnecessary surgery. If your hips are generous, you might want to consider having both procedures.

Tummy Tuck: The Operation

As stated earlier, a tummy tuck is major surgery. There are several ways to perform it. The most common technique is called "full tummy tuck" or "full abdominoplasty" and involves four steps (fig. 9-3):

1. removing most of the skin and fat between your belly button and your pubic hair in a horizontal oval;
2. tightening the fascia with permanent sutures (some surgeons may refer to this as "tightening the muscle," but they are actually tightening the fascia, which overlies the abdominal muscles);
3. repositioning your belly button (your belly button does not actually move, but the skin surrounding it does); and
4. sewing together the remaining skin above your pubic hair.

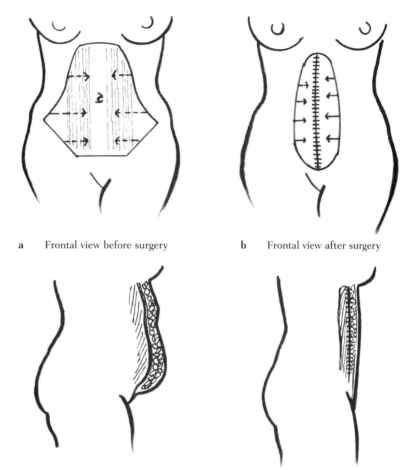

a   Frontal view before surgery   b   Frontal view after surgery

c   Profile view before surgery   d   Profile view after surgery

FIGURE 9-3: *Tummy tuck. (a) Before surgery, the skin is lifted up, showing the fascia under-neath. The muscles are widely separated. Arrows show the direction the fascia will be pulled together and tightened. (b) After surgery a zipperlike seam is shown where the fascia has been sewn together and tightened. The waist is narrowed, and the abdomen appears flat. (c) Before surgery the fascia is lax and skin is loose. (d) After surgery, the tightened fascia no longer bows forward.*

Incisions and Scars

Scars are designed to fall along natural skin creases within the bikini line. Scar length is variable. Scars may be limited to the pubic area in thin women but may extend beyond the hips in large women. The final visibility of scars varies significantly from person to person. Your scar may be almost invisible or may be wide and unsightly. Your final scar depends on your healing characteristics, but it can also be affected by how tightly your incision was closed. If your belly button was repositioned, there will be a scar around it. In addition, there may

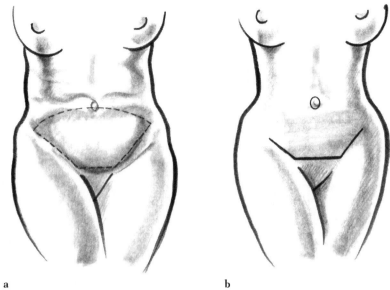

a   b

FIGURE 9-4: *Tummy tuck incision and scars. (a) The skin to be removed (dashed line). (b) The scars will be around the belly button and in the bikini line (solid lines). The waist is narrower.*

be a small vertical scar just above your pubic hair if all lower abdominal skin could not be removed. This vertical scar corresponds to the previous skin location of your belly button (fig. 9-4).

Modified Techniques

1. *Mini tummy tuck.* This procedure removes loose skin of the lower abdomen but does not reposition the belly button or tighten upper abdomen loose skin. It may or may not tighten the fascia. It is best suited to thin women with firm inner girdles and moderately loose lower abdominal skin. Mini tummy tuck uses shorter incisions and avoids scars around the belly button.

2. *Endoscopic tummy tuck.* In this technique, your surgeon uses an endoscope to tighten your fascia but does not remove skin. Liposuction of the abdomen may be more thorough than with the other techniques because the incision is small and so blood supply is less interrupted for healing. Scar length is only a few inches. This operation is best for women with lax fascia but no loose skin. Because most women with lax fascia also have loose skin, this technique is rarely used.

Vital Statistics

Tummy Tuck

Anesthesia: General or heavy sedation.

Location of operation: Office or hospital.

Length of surgery: 1–3 hours.

Length of stay: Overnight for pain control.

Discomfort: Moderate to severe. The tighter your surgeon makes your fascia, the greater your discomfort will be. Anticipate 3–14 days of prescription pain medication.

Swelling: Will peak in 3 days. Most swelling will improve within 2–4 weeks but may take 3 months to improve completely. As it resolves, it will linger in your lower abdomen above your scar line and may temporarily make this area look unnaturally full.

Bruising: Does not usually occur.

Numbness: Abdominal numbness is expected and may last for 6 months or longer. If numbness is persistent, you will get used to it. Most do not find this bothersome.

Bandages: Removed in 2–4 days.

Stitches: Most plastic surgeons use absorbable stitches under the skin that do not require removal. If your surgeon uses nonabsorbable stitches, they will be visible and will be removed in 7 days.

Drains: Will be placed at the time of surgery to prevent postoperative fluid collections, called "seromas." The drain tubes are plastic and will be connected to small reservoirs the size of tennis balls. You will go home with drains and will be instructed to empty them several times daily. Your surgeon will remove your drains between 2 days and 2 weeks following surgery. The drains are not painful, but their removal causes temporary discomfort.

Support: You may be given an abdominal binder following surgery. It is a broad elastic band that should be worn continuously for 2–6 weeks. The binder will provide extra comfort and support as you heal.

Presentable in a bathing suit: Your abdomen will immediately look better in most one-piece bathing suits than it did prior to surgery. However, a two-piece bathing suit may not conceal your scars. You may need to choose your swimwear carefully. If your scar is exposed while you are outdoors, you should protect it with sunscreen SPF 15 or higher for at least one year to prevent discoloration. You must also avoid tanning beds.

Work: You may return to work once you have stopped taking prescription pain medication. For most, this is 1–2 weeks. If your job requires lifting or manual labor, wait 4–6 weeks.

Driving: May be resumed in 7–14 days, if you have stopped taking prescription pain medication.

Exercise: May be resumed in 4 weeks.

Final result: Is seen after your scar has matured, approximately 1 year.

3. *Conservative abdominal liposuction with full tummy tuck.* This procedure is performed by some surgeons and is most appropriate for women who desire conservative liposuction of their upper abdomens and flanks. Because of possible healing complications, as noted previously, thorough abdominal liposuction should not be performed at the same time as a full tummy tuck.

What to Expect

Tummy tucks are commonly performed under general anesthesia, and recovery is similar to that following a C-section. Your surgeon will probably recommend that you stay overnight for pain control. Discomfort is moderate to severe and is usually controlled with intravenous pain medication for the first 24 hours followed by prescription oral pain medication at home. You will be able to return to sedentary work in one to two weeks and may resume exercise in four weeks.

To help you to plan for and recover from your procedure, reread Steps 7 and 10 of Chapter 1.

Complications

When your operation is performed by a qualified plastic surgeon, both your procedure and recovery will likely be uneventful. Even in ideal circumstances, however, complications may occur. In addition to the specific complications mentioned here, refer to Chapter 1 for general complications that may follow any procedure.

Skin Death

If skin death occurs, it usually involves the skin above your pubic hair. Depending on the size of the affected area, it may heal on its own within a few weeks or may require further surgery. Skin death may occur in anyone, but is more likely if you smoke, have poorly controlled diabetes, have had previous abdominal surgery, or are overweight. All of these factors compromise circulation to the skin and confound healing. If you are at high risk for skin death, your surgeon may either advise against tummy tuck or may choose to remove less skin

When Can I Stop Worrying About Complications?

Most complications occur within a predictable time following surgery. If you do not develop them within the time periods noted, you can fairly conclude that you are probably free of these complications.

TIME	AFTER	POSSBILE COMPLICATIONS
2 weeks	Drain removal	Seroma
2 weeks	Surgery	Skin death
2 weeks	Surgery	Belly button death
2 weeks	Surgery	Hematoma
3 weeks	Surgery	Infection
4 weeks	Surgery	Seroma
2 months	Surgery	Suture rupture

so what remains is closed without tension, to ease circulation. If the latter is chosen, your aesthetic outcome may be compromised.

Infection

Infection may occur and may require hospitalization, intravenous antibiotics, and further surgery. Infection is uncommon unless skin death occurs.

Hematoma

A *hematoma* is a collection of blood under the skin. If it develops, it usually does so within a day of surgery. Even if identified and treated quickly, it may block circulation enough to cause skin death. Hematomas following tummy tuck usually require an operation for removal.

Seroma

A *seroma* is a collection of fluid under your skin. Drainage tubes are used to prevent seromas, but they may occur anyway. Seroma fluid can be removed by your surgeon in the office through a needle and syringe. This is not painful, because your abdominal skin will be numb for several months following tummy tuck. Sometimes, fluid requires repeated removal. Seroma accumulation is one of the most common problems following tummy tuck, but it does not usually alter the final cosmetic result.

Suture Rupture

If the suture that tightens your inner girdle breaks, you may rapidly redevelop lax fascia. Correction requires reoperation with placement of a new suture. The risk of suture rupture is minimized by avoiding abdominal strain during the first four weeks after surgery.

Belly Button Death

Your belly button skin may lose its circulation and die. If this happens, the area develops a scar. Because a normal belly button resembles a scar, the new scar is usually cosmetically acceptable.

Reasons to Avoid or Postpone a Tummy Tuck

Future Pregnancies

Defer your tummy tuck until you are done childbearing. If you bear children following tummy tuck, you may require another operation to correct recurrent fascia laxity and loose skin.

Previous Abdominal Scars

If you have extensive horizontal scars across your upper abdomen, you are at high risk for healing problems. Your surgeon will probably advise against tummy tuck.

Obesity

If you are obese, the circulation to your abdominal skin and fat may be too poor for proper healing following tummy tuck. You will be at high risk for skin death, infection, and wound separation. If you are obese and have droopy skin, a better approach may be *panniculectomy.* That involves removal of droopy skin and fat of the lower abdomen, without tightening the fascia. Panniculectomy is sometimes covered by insurance if your excess skin causes back pain or hygiene problems.

Smoking

If you smoke, you have a greatly increased risk of healing problems, and you will be advised to quit before surgery. If you are unable to quit, your surgeon may cancel your surgery or may choose to remove less skin than would be considered optimal.

Breast Cancer

If your mother or sister had breast cancer, you are at higher than average risk for developing it yourself. Even if no family members have had breast cancer, your lifetime risk is one in nine. Breast cancer is sometimes treated with breast removal, also called mastectomy. If reconstruction after mastectomy is desired, the most common technique for breast reconstruction is called a TRAM flap, which uses abdominal skin and fat. If you have a tummy tuck, you cannot later have this type of breast reconstruction. (Few physicians consider this a valid reason to avoid tummy tuck because: you may never get breast cancer, you may not need mastectomy if you do, and other options are available for breast reconstruction.)

Telltale Signs

Scars

You may have a visible scar around your belly button. Your belly button may also become distorted. Your scar may be visible in swimwear—even in a one-piece bathing suit.

Dog Ears

Puckered skin, called a "dog ear," may occur on either end of the scar, because there is always more skin above the suture line than below it. (Puckering can usually be avoided if your surgeon gathers the upper skin in the middle or extends the incision to your hip bones.) If your surgeon originally recommended a total body lift, but you chose to have only a tummy tuck, expect dog ears. They may be removed through an office procedure.

Pubic Hair Lift

The upper border of your pubic hair will be lifted following tummy tuck. This is not usually a problem unless you wear low-cut bikinis. However, if your pubic hair is raised significantly, your vaginal opening may also be pulled forward. This may cause pain during intercourse. Further surgery may improve this problem, but, depending on its severity, may not resolve it. Fortunately, this problem is uncommon.

Cost

In the United States, the range of total fees for a tummy tuck extends from $5,000 to $8,000. The average cost is:

Surgeon's fee	$ 4,300
Anesthesiologist's fee	$ 700
Operating room fee	$ 1,000
Hospital fee for overnight stay	$ 500
Total	**$6,500**

See "Fees" in Chapter 1 for various factors that might affect your own actual cost.

Duration of Results

Within six months of tummy tuck, your newly tightened inner girdle may loosen slightly. It will remain stable thereafter. Unless you become pregnant or gain substantial weight, your tummy tuck results should be lasting.

Satisfaction

Patient satisfaction following surgery is high if expectations are realistic and complications are avoided.

Concluding Thoughts

Women with excess skin or lax fascia may try diet and exercise, only to discover that weight loss and improved muscle tone do not solve these problems. Tummy tuck offers these women an opportunity to regain the tighter, flatter abdomen they had in youth—but not without risk. Tummy tuck is a deceptively innocuous name for a major operation. Recovery is not easy and potential complications are serious. As long as these issues are fully understood, tummy tuck can be a gratifying procedure.

Inner Thigh Lift

Inner thigh lift, also called medial thigh lift, was designed for women with sagging inner thigh skin. Standing in front of a mirror, use your thumb and forefinger to pinch the skin of your inner thigh near your groin. Now, lift it upward. This will show you the effect of an inner thigh lift. If you have loose, excess inner thigh skin, you may be a candidate for this operation.

Lift Versus Liposuction

It has been said that liposuction will make one look thinner, while a lift will make one look younger. An inner thigh lift will remove loose skin and lift the remaining skin. Liposuction will reduce fat volume, but may worsen the appearance of your inner thighs if your primary problem is skin laxity.

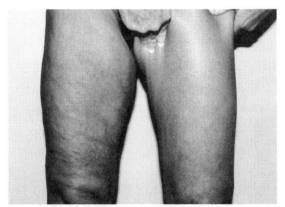

When this woman lifts the loose skin of her left thigh, her cellulite improves. This demonstrates the potential effect an inner thigh lift may have on her.

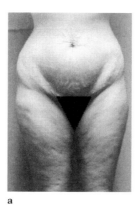
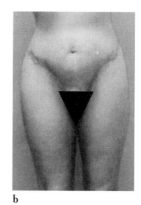

a   b

(a) Before inner thigh lift. (b) After inner thigh lift; this woman also had a tummy tuck and lipo-
suction of her outer thighs.

Reprinted with permission from Ted Lockwood, M.D., "Superficial Fascial System Suspension," *Plastic*
and Reconstructive Surgery, 92(6):1112–1122.

Loose inner thigh skin typically has poor tone; thus it will not reliably contract following liposuction. If your main problem is loose skin, an inner thigh
lift is the procedure for you. If your problem is both loose skin and excess fat,
you may attempt liposuction and hope for some skin tightening. Understand,
however, that inner thigh lift may be necessary, also. Some plastic surgeons
perform inner thigh lift and liposuction together. Others do not, because of
the increased risk of healing complications.

Inner Thigh Lift Procedure

An inner thigh lift removes loose skin and anchors remaining skin to your
pubic bone area. Your scar should be in your groin crease and will hopefully
heal undetectably (fig. 9-5).

What to Expect

Inner thigh lifts are commonly performed under general anesthesia. Your surgeon may recommend that you stay overnight. Discomfort is moderate and
will be controlled with prescription pain medication. You will be able to return
to sedentary work within one to two weeks and may slowly resume exercise
in four weeks.

To help you to plan for and recover from your procedure, reread Steps 7
and 10 of Chapter 1.

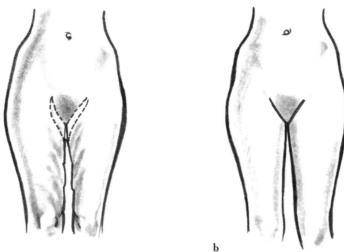

a   b

FIGURE 9-5: *Inner thigh lift. (a) The incisions (dashed lines). (b) The scars within the groin creases (solid lines).*

Vital Statistics

INNER THIGH LIFT

Anesthesia: *General.*

Location of operation: *Office or hospital.*

Length of surgery: *1–2 hours.*

Length of stay: *Overnight.*

Discomfort: *Moderate. Anticipate 2–7 days of prescription pain medication.*

Swelling: *Will peak at 3 days. As thigh swelling improves, you may notice swelling in your knees and ankles. All swelling should improve within 2–6 weeks. Keep your legs elevated to expedite this process.*

Bruising: *Improves in 5–10 days. If liposuction is not also performed, there may be no bruising.*

Bandages: *Removed in 2–4 days.*

Stitches: *Most plastic surgeons use absorbable stitches that do not require removal. If your surgeon uses non-absorbable stitches, they will be removed in 7–10 days.*

Drains: *If drains are placed, they will be removed in 1–3 days.*

Presentable in a bathing suit: *2 weeks.*

Work: *You may return to sedentary work in 1–2 weeks, if you have stopped taking prescription pain medication. If you are able to keep your feet elevated at work, you may return sooner.*

Driving: *May be resumed in 1–2 weeks, if you have stopped taking prescription pain medication.*

Exercise: *May be gradually resumed in 4 weeks.*

Final result: *Is seen after your scars have matured, approximately 6 months.*

Complications

When your operation is performed by a qualified plastic surgeon, both your procedure and recovery will likely be uneventful. Even in ideal circumstances, however, complications may occur. In addition to the specific complications mentioned here, refer to Chapter 1 for general complications that may follow any procedure.

Healing Complications

Healing problems may lead to infection or wound separation. If so, you may require hospitalization and intravenous antibiotics. (Fortunately, most wound problems are relatively minor.) Healing problems are more common in smokers and diabetics. If the surgeon removed too much skin or closed it too tightly, healing complications are also more likely.

Baggy Skin

If your surgeon did not remove enough skin, droopiness will persist. Reoperation to remove more skin can remedy this problem.

Sensory Changes

Numbness and tingling of your inner thigh may occur temporarily. Numbness may be permanent if the sensory nerve was cut or damaged during surgery. If so, it will be quite bothersome for six to twelve months. Thereafter, you may get used to it.

Downward Drift of Your Scar

If the anchoring sutures rupture or if too much skin was removed, your scars may descend onto your thigh. Then they will no longer be hidden in your groin creases. Worse, your vaginal opening may be widened, often causing pain during intercourse, persistent discomfort, or both.

Cases in which the anchoring sutures ruptured may be improved through re-anchoring of thigh skin to the pubic bone. If too much skin was removed, the problem may be difficult to remedy through further surgery.

When Can I Stop Worrying About Complications?

Most complications occur within a predictable time following surgery. If you do not develop them within the time periods noted, you can fairly conclude that you are probably free of these complications.

Time After Surgery	Possible Complication
2 weeks	*Poor healing or infection*
2 weeks	*Sensory changes*
4 weeks	*Persistent bagginess*
4 weeks	*Persistent swelling*
3 months	*Downward drift of the scar*

Telltale Signs

Scars are the telltale signs of inner thigh lift. They may be visible in some swimwear, especially if they drift downward.

Cost

In the United States, the range of total fees for an inner thigh lift extends from $4,000 to $6,000. The average cost is:

Surgeon's fee	$3,400
Anesthesiologist's fee	$ 700
Operating room (facility) fee	$ 900
Total	$5,000

See "Fees" in Chapter 1 for various factors that might affect your own actual cost.

Duration of Results

Your newly tightened inner thigh skin will loosen slowly in response to gravity. In 10 years, you may be ready for another inner thigh lift. If you lose weight, your skin may become lax, and you may be ready for another lift sooner.

Satisfaction

Because diet and exercise will not improve loose inner thigh skin, women who suffer from this problem become frustrated. If and when they choose to proceed with inner thigh lift, they are highly gratified. Usually, the greater their sagginess before surgery, the more they are rewarded afterward.

Concluding Thoughts

Inner thigh lift offers the potential to reduce baggy inner thigh skin and restore a more youthful appearance. It is, however, a major operation with significant medical risks.

Outer Thigh and Buttock Lift

Outer thigh and buttock lift was designed for women with sagging skin in these areas. Standing in front of a mirror, place one hand on the outside of each thigh at the level of your hip and lift upward. This demonstrates the effects of an outer thigh lift. Now, with your back to the mirror, hold a hand mirror so that you can see your buttocks. Place your remaining hand above one buttock at the hip level and lift it up. This will show you the effect of a buttock lift. If you have cellulite, you may find that lifting your thighs and buttocks improves it.

Cellulite

Your droopy skin is tethered by inelastic fibers to your bone. In some people, the skin around the fibers droops over time, which creates the puckering we call "cellulite." (Most people believe it is due solely to fat, but it is not that simple. Cellulite is due to a combination of fat, fibrous tissue, and gravity.)

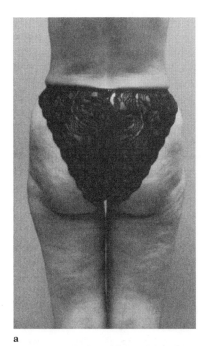 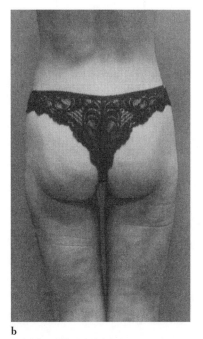

a   b

(a) Before outer thigh and buttock lift. (b) After outer thigh and buttock lift.

Reprinted with permission from Ted Lockwood, M.D., "Superficial Fascial System Suspension," *Plastic and Reconstructive Surgery*, 92(6):1112–1122.

An outer thigh and buttock lift may take tension off the tethered fibers and relieve skin puckering.

When you perform your self-evaluation in front of a mirror, note whether you have cellulite. If you do, pay attention to whether it improves while you lift your thigh and buttock skin. If it does, it may also improve following a thigh and buttock lift. Even so, be guarded in your expectations.

Outer Thigh and Buttock Lift Procedure

Outer thigh lift and buttock lift are usually performed as one procedure. Prior to surgery, your surgeon will mark the areas of skin to be removed (fig. 9-6). After removal of loose skin, the remaining skin will be pulled upward and anchored in position with sutures. If you have excess fat in addition to droopy skin, your surgeon may recommend liposuction. Most surgeons will leave drain tubes under your skin at the completion of surgery.

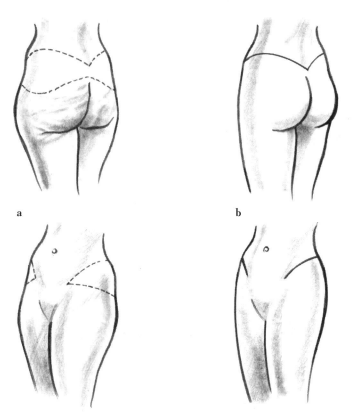

a   b

FIGURE 9-6: *Outer thigh and buttock lift. (a) The incisions (dashed lines). The area between the dashed lines is the skin to be removed. (b) The position of the resulting scars (solid lines).*

Incisions and Scars

Following this operation, you will look better in clothing and in most swimwear. When you are unclothed, however, your scar will be obvious. It will extend from hip to hip across the top of your buttocks (fig. 9-6 b, right). The final appearance of your scar is difficult to predict. Your scar may fade and flatten, or it may widen and become unsightly. Do not expect this scar to become invisible; it does not heal as well as scars in other areas. It should be hidden by a one-piece bathing suit, but it may be visible in a bikini. Even if your scar is initially below your bikini line, it may migrate up or down in response to gravity or skin tension.

What to Expect

Outer thigh and buttock lifts are most commonly performed under general anesthesia. Your surgeon will recommend an overnight stay for

---

Vital Statistics

Outer Thigh and Buttock Lift

Anesthesia: General.

Location of operation: Office or hospital.

Length of surgery: 2–4 hours.

Length of stay: 1–2 nights.

Discomfort: Moderate to severe. Anticipate 5–14 days of prescription pain medication.

Swelling: Improves in 2–4 weeks.

Bandages: Removed in 2–4 days.

Stitches: Most plastic surgeons use absorbable stitches that do not require removal. Nonabsorbable stitches will be removed in 7–10 days.

Drains: If drains are placed, they will be removed in 1–3 days.

Presentable in a bathing suit: 2–4 weeks. Be certain to wear sunscreen (SPF 15–40) for at least one year on any scars that may be exposed to sun.

Work: You will be able to return to work in 1–3 weeks, if you have stopped taking prescription pain medication. If your job requires lifting, you should wait 4 weeks.

Driving: May be resumed in 2 weeks, if you have stopped taking prescription pain medication.

Exercise: May be resumed in 4–6 weeks.

Final result: Will be seen after scar maturation, approximately 1 year.

observation and pain control. Discomfort is moderate to severe and will be controlled with intravenous pain medication for the first 24 hours. You will also need prescription pain medication at home. You will be able to return to sedentary work in about two weeks and may resume exercise within six weeks.

To help you to plan for and recover from your procedure reread Steps 7 and 10 of Chapter 1.

Complications

When your operation is performed by a qualified plastic surgeon, both your procedure and recovery will likely be uneventful. Even in ideal circumstances, however, complications may occur. The risks described for inner thigh lift also apply to outer thigh and buttock lift. The risk of healing complications and infections are higher for outer thigh and buttock lift.

Telltale Sign

The scar is a telltale sign for outer thigh and buttock lift. Scarring is the greatest drawback of this procedure.

Cost

In the United States, the range of total fees for an outer thigh and buttock lift extends from $5,000 to $8,000. The average cost is:

Surgeon's fee	$ 4,000
Anesthesiologist's fee	$ 800
Operating room (facility) fee	$ 1,200
Hospital fee for overnight stay	$ 500
Total	$ 6,500

See "Fees" in Chapter 1 for various factors that might affect your own actual cost.

GWEN, *a 53-year-old socialite with a flamboyant personality, grabbed her buttocks in the exam room, pulled them up, and exclaimed, "I need this lifted." She wanted an outer thigh and buttock lift, which we proceeded to discuss. As I rose to leave, she said, "Oh, and I need this tucked, too," as she grabbed her lower abdomen, pinched it together, and pulled it outward. We proceeded to discuss tummy tuck. As I again began to exit, she stopped me, pulled her inner thigh skin up, and said, " Can you do this, too?" A total body lift was born.*

Duration of Results

Your newly tightened outer thighs and buttocks will slowly descend in response to gravity. In 10 years, you may be ready for another lift.

Satisfaction

Satisfaction following surgery is closely tied to the degree of droop before surgery. So, if your droop is mild before surgery, you may be unimpressed with your result and unhappy with your scars. If your droop is moderate to severe, you will most likely be pleased with your result and consider the procedure worthwhile.

Concluding Thoughts

Outer thigh and buttock lift can lift droopy buttocks and restore more youthful contours to outer thighs. Some women also gain an improvement in cellulite. If you seek this procedure, you must be prepared for major surgery and extensive scars. In the end, you will probably be pleased with your choice and satisfied with your new appearance.

Total Body Lift (Lower Body Lift)

A total body lift, also called "lower body lift," includes tummy tuck, inner thigh lift, and outer thigh and buttock lift (fig. 9-7). Surgery is extensive; however, the results are gratifying. The procedure may take five to eight hours and mandate a one- to three-night hospital stay. Blood loss may be enough to merit transfusion. (You may choose to donate your own blood a few weeks prior to surgery. If you need a transfusion, you will then receive your own blood.) You may return to sedentary work in three to six weeks.

Because a total body lift entails having tummy tuck, inner thigh lift, and outer thigh and buttock lift at the same time, the risks applicable to

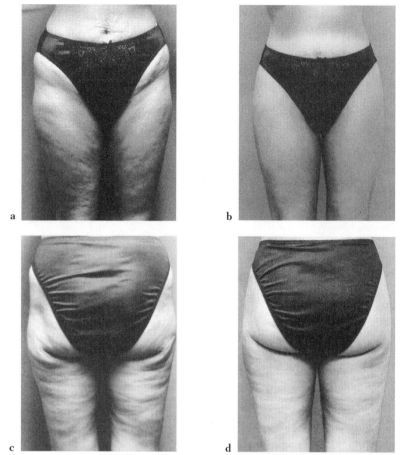

(a and c) Before total body lift. (b and d) After total body lift.

Reprinted with permission from Ted Lockwood, M.D., "Superficial Fascial System Suspension," *Plastic and Reconstructive Surgery*, 92(6):1112–1122.

all components must be considered, and the recovery is lengthy. You and your surgeon should decide together if you are a candidate for this procedure, or if you should undergo each component separately to minimize risk. Given the magnitude of this operation, some surgeons advise performing it in stages.

Cost

In the United States, the range of total fees for a total body lift extends from $8,000 to $20,000. The average cost is:

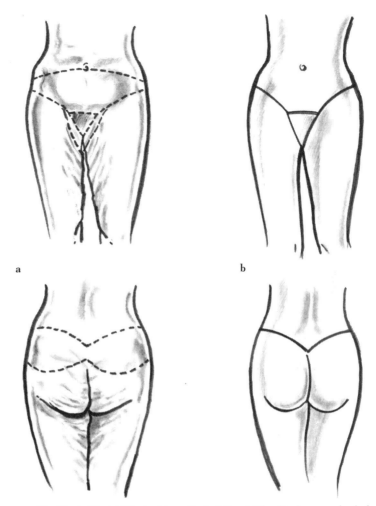

FIGURE 9-7: *Total body lift. (a) The incisions (dashed lines). The skin between the dashed lines will be removed. (b) The resultant scars (solid lines). A total body lift is the combination of a tummy tuck, inner thigh lift, and outer thigh and buttock lift.*

Surgeon's fee	$ 10,000
Anesthesiologist's fee	$ 1,500
Operating room (facility) fee	$ 2,000
Hospital fee for overnight stay	$ 1,000
Total	**$14,500**

See "Fees" in Chapter 1 for various factors that might affect your own actual cost. For example, if you plan to have this procedure in New York, expect to pay an average of $20,000 in total fees with a range from $15,000 to 25,000.

Concluding Thoughts

Total body lift is a serious operation. Do not underestimate the enormity of this procedure. You must be prepared for extensive surgery and lengthy recovery. If you proceed, you must keep these issues in mind and be willing to accept potential complications. If you do have this procedure and emerge without complications, you will probably be satisfied.

Questions to Ask Your Plastic Surgeon

Will my cellulite be improved?

Will you be able to remove my stretch marks?

Where will my scars be?

Tips and Traps

Diet and exercise alone will not tighten your loose skin.

If you seek tummy tuck, wait until you have finished childbearing.

If you have a tummy tuck, then your abdominal tissue will not be available for future breast reconstruction. This is relevant only if you later require mastectomy for breast cancer.

If your hips are wide, consider hip liposuction at the same time as tummy tuck.

If you have thick abdominal fat, lax skin, and loose fascia, your surgeon may recommend both tummy tuck and abdominal liposuction as separate operations at 6-month intervals.

Beware a surgeon who advocates thorough abdominal liposuction at the same time as tummy tuck. This can disrupt circulation and predispose you to healing problems.

Thigh lift and buttock lift may or may not improve cellulite.

If you smoke, have poorly controlled diabetes, or are overweight, you will be at significantly increased risk for complications.

10

Defining Body Contour

Liposuction

MANDY, *a 24-year-old sales representative, was proud of her diligent diet and exercise. Despite her attractive body, she was self-conscious around her apartment swimming pool because of her large thighs. Regardless of her effort, she could not trim them down. She initially resisted liposuction, because she thought it was for those who were too lazy to diet and exercise. Eventually, when she saw no improvement from her strict regime, she underwent liposuction. Following thigh liposuction, she was more comfortable around the pool, and she more easily found clothes that fit. She continues her healthy diet and exercise and now encourages others with diet-resistant fat to consider liposuction.*

*L*iposuction is the most popular cosmetic procedure performed in the United States. The problem of localized fatty deposits affects women of all ages. Contrary to popular opinion, those who seek liposuction commonly follow vigorous diet and exercise programs. However, they remain unable to lose fat in specific areas such as the hips or outer thighs. Liposuction can safely and effectively remove this diet-resistant fat.

Most of this chapter discusses both basic questions and sophisticated concerns regarding liposuction in general. The last part of this chapter compares and contrasts the three types of liposuction (traditional, ultrasonic, and external ultrasound–assisted).

Fat Facts

You are born with a genetically determined number of fat cells. Throughout childhood and adolescence, the size and number of your fat cells increase, even if you remain at ideal body weight for your height

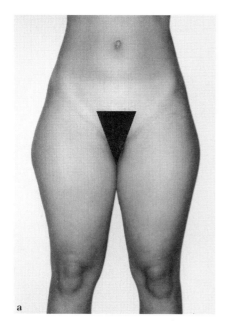
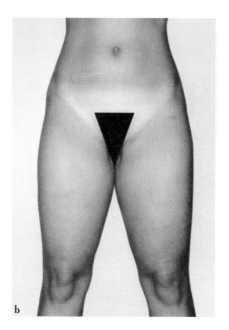
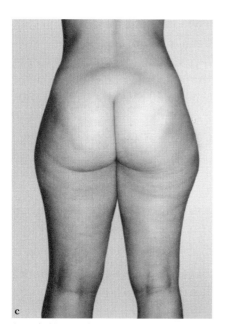
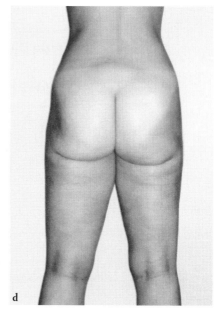

(a and c) Before liposuction of the outer thighs. (b and d) After liposuction of the outer thighs.

and age. After adolescence, any fat accumulation will increase fat-cell size. But new fat cells are not formed unless you approach morbid obesity (twice your ideal body weight).

Candidates for Liposuction

The best candidates for liposuction are those who are near their ideal body weight but have fat deposits that are resistant to diet and exercise. For those who are slightly or moderately overweight, liposuction can provide incentive for weight loss. Liposuction alone, however, is not a method of weight control. It is no substitute for diet and exercise.

KAREN, *a 39-year-old data entry specialist, sought evaluation for liposuction. She said that her metabolism had changed, and she was gaining weight. Her weight had recently increased by 15 pounds, and she continued to slowly gain. Diet and exercise had not helped. She was certain that liposuction would solve her problems. However, I told her that she was not a good candidate for liposuction because of her recent pattern of weight gain. She sought a second opinion and proceeded with liposuction through that surgeon. She was initially pleased but continued her steady weight gain. Not surprisingly, one year later, she weighed even more and was frustrated with her previous decision to have liposuction.*

Not for Obesity

Liposuction is not a treatment for obesity. True, if you seek liposuction for weight control, you will likely find a doctor who is willing to perform the procedure. Unfortunately, you are unlikely to have a pleasing or lasting result.

Requires a Steady Weight

The best time to consider liposuction is after you have stabilized your weight through diet and exercise. If you have diet-resistant fat deposits and your weight has been stable for 6 to 12 months, then you will probably be a good candidate for liposuction.

If you have been gaining weight prior to surgery, you most likely will continue to gain weight and develop new fat deposits in the area treated with liposuction.

If you have been losing weight, you should wait until it has stabilized. Otherwise, you may undergo unnecessary liposuction in some areas.

Good Skin Tone

Having good skin tone is one of the keys to attractive results following liposuction. The better the skin's tone the better it will contract to fit the newly contoured fat following surgery. Several factors influence skin tone:

Good Skin Tone	Poor Skin Tone
Tight skin	Loose skin
Younger patients	Older patients
Thick skin, such as outer thighs	Thin skin, such as inner thighs
Stretch marks absent	Stretch marks present
Minimal prior sun exposure	Extensive prior sun exposure

Thus, a young woman seeking treatment of her outer thighs will have better results than an older woman seeking treatment of her inner thighs. But a 35-year-old woman with tight inner thigh skin may still have acceptable results. And a 20-year-old woman with stretch marks on her outer thighs may have poor results. All five factors affecting skin tone must be taken into account.

Best Body Areas for Liposuction

Certain areas of the body have good skin tone in nearly all women (fig. 10-1, speckled areas). These include the outer thighs, hips, knees, flanks, back, and neck. Thus, these areas tend to show good liposuction results.

Body Areas That Yield Mixed Results

Not all body areas are equally amenable to liposuction (fig. 10-1, cross-hatched areas). Some areas will yield favorable results only if skin tone happens to be good. Likewise, areas with only superficial fat, such as the calves, will yield satisfactory results only under certain conditions. And areas with natural skin creases, such as the buttock crease, are likely to yield poor results unless certain conditions are met.

Areas with Poor Skin Tone

Where skin is loose and thin, it will fail to tighten after liposuction—and it may appear looser and baggier. In these cases, removal of excess skin is more appropriate than liposuction. For example, women with poor skin tone of their inner thighs may get a better result following inner thigh lift than liposuction. Similarly, loose abdominal skin with stretch marks will not contract well following abdominal liposuction; women with these skin features should instead consider tummy tuck.

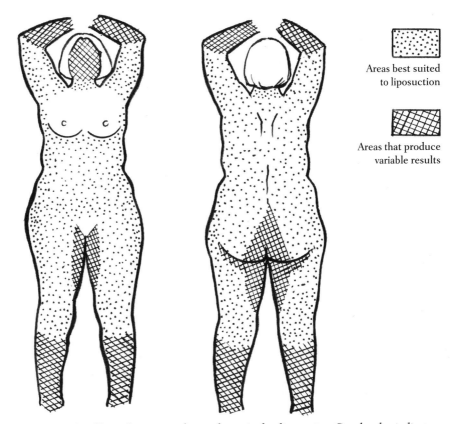

Areas best suited
to liposuction

Areas that produce
variable results

FIGURE 10-1: *Speckles indicate areas that are best suited to liposuction. Crosshatches indicate areas where liposuction results vary.*

Areas with Only Superficial Fat

Most areas of the body have two layers of fat: a thin, superficial layer and a thicker, deep layer. Liposuction is primarily aimed at removing deep fat, because suction of superficial fat may lead to skin irregularities, dimpling, and puckering.

The calves, unlike other areas of the body, have only a superficial layer of fat. Therefore, calf liposuction risks causing the problems just mentioned. Yet when performed by an experienced plastic surgeon, it can be safe and effective. Calf liposuction also leads to marked swelling. Bed rest and leg elevation are mandatory for several weeks following surgery, which most women consider impractical.

Likewise, the face has only superficial fat and is prone to dimpling and irregularities following liposuction. Most surgeons avoid liposuction of the face, because the results have generally been poor.

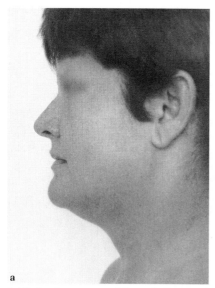 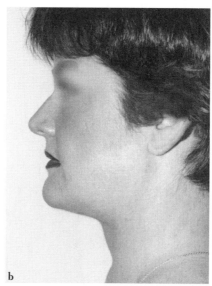

a   b

(a) Before liposuction of the neck. (b) After liposuction of the neck.

A minority of surgeons do perform superficial liposuction routinely. Presumably they have extensive experience with it and have not found an increased risk of complications. If you seek superficial liposuction, choose a surgeon with experience in this technique. Ask how many superficial liposuction procedures your surgeon has performed. (Superficial liposuction is further discussed in the section on cellulite.)

Areas with Natural Creases

Liposuction of the crease between the buttock and thigh can disrupt the fibrous bands between skin and bone that maintain the crease. If so, this causes the buttock to droop. Therefore, most surgeons avoid liposuction of the buttock crease.

A noteworthy exception is the fat roll, often called the banana roll, immediately below the buttock crease. Delicately performed liposuction here will not disrupt the fibrous bands above it.

Liposuction Versus Other Surgery

Lift

Inner thighs, outer thighs, and buttocks may lend themselves to either liposuction or lift. Sometimes it is difficult to know which technique will yield the best results. If your problem involves loose skin with poor tone, lift will be best. If your problem is excess fat, then liposuction is most appropriate. In general, liposuction will make you look thinner, whereas a lift will make you look younger. (See Chapter 9 for more information on lifts.)

Tummy Tuck

Many women with flabby abdomens seek liposuction. Liposuction, however, does not always yield much improvement. This is because your abdomen's appearance depends on more than just fat. Your skin and inner girdle are also factors. The inner girdle is a sheet of tough connective tissue. It extends from your ribs down to your pubic bone, and it functions to keep your internal organs inside your abdomen. After being stretched during pregnancy, it often fails to regain tone. For women with lax inner girdles or loose skin, tummy tuck is better suited than liposuction. (See Chapter 9 for a self-assessment to determine your needs.)

Hips and Thighs

Harmony in the Body Contour

Standing unclothed in front of a full-length mirror, examine the outline of your body. If the outline of your flank, hip, and outer thigh follow one smooth, gentle curve around your frame, then you probably do not need body liposuction. If your silhouette bulges outward at your hips and again at your thighs, then liposuction may be appropriate. Bulging hips and thighs cast a cellolike silhouette (fig. 10-2).

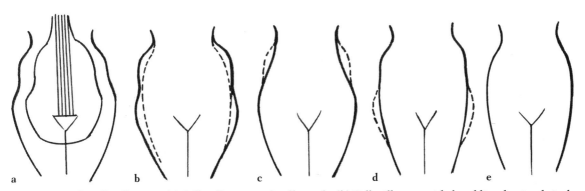

FIGURE 10-2: *The cello silhouette. (a) Cello silhouette with cello inside. (b) Cello silhouette with dotted line showing desired contour. The depression between hips and thighs should not be suctioned. (c) Cello silhouette following liposuction of hips only. Wide thighs appear wider. (d) Cello silhouette following liposuction of the thighs alone. Wide hips appear wider. (e) Silhouette following liposuction of hips and thighs.*

If you have a cello silhouette and get liposuction of your hips alone, your outer thighs may look larger by comparison. If you get liposuction of your outer thighs alone, then your hips may look larger by comparison (fig. 10-2). The best result will be obtained by suctioning both hips and outer thighs—but not the depression between them—to bring your entire contour into harmony.

Avoiding Natural Depressions

Surgeons avoid performing liposuction in areas of natural concavity, such as the natural depression between your outer thigh and hip. Avoiding these areas allows your surgeon to bring your hips and outer thighs into alignment with these depressions. Otherwise, the "cello" appearance may persist (fig. 10-3).

Cellulite

Cellulite is a common but unattractive dimpling and puckering of the skin. Unfortunately, it is not improved through liposuction.

Cellulite is caused by a combination of fibrous bands and superficial fat. Inelastic fibrous bands connect the skin and deep layer of fat, passing through the superficial layer of fat. When superficial fat compartments become distended with fat, fibrous bands tether the skin, causing dimpling

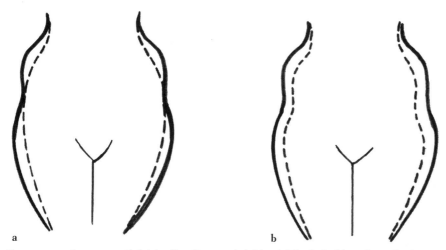

a   b

FIGURE 10-3: *Areas to avoid. (a) A cello silhouette (solid line). The dashed line shows the desired contour. The depression between hips and thighs needs no liposuction to accomplish the desired result. (b) After liposuction of the depression is performed along with liposuction of the hips and thighs: a smaller cello results.*

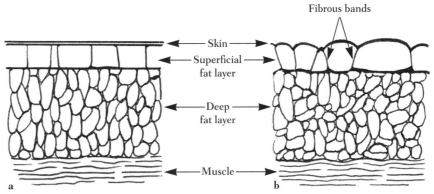

FIGURE 10-4: *Cellulite. (a) Superficial and deep fat layers without cellulite. (b) The superficial layer of fat becomes distended, causing the fat to bulge around the skin-tethering bands. This creates the dimpled appearance of cellulite.*

KELLY, *a 33-year-old industrial engineer, was troubled by cellulite of her buttocks and thighs. When she learned that liposuction would not improve her cellulite she was surprised. After she discovered that weight gain following liposuction might worsen her cellulite, she wisely chose not to proceed.*

at the points of attachment (fig. 10-4). Cellulite only occurs in the areas that have fibrous bands, such as the buttocks and thighs.

To remove cellulite through liposuction, your plastic surgeon would have to suction the superficial layer of fat. Superficial liposuction, however, is fraught with increased risks of skin death, dimpling, puckering, and irregularity. These complications are difficult to correct. The few surgeons who do perform superficial liposuction take those chances in the hope for better skin retraction and reduced cellulite. But neither presumed benefit has been proved.

No consistently good treatment for cellulite exists, although some surgeons have reduced cellulite with outer thigh/buttock lift or endermologie. (Refer to Chapters 9 and 13 for more information on these procedures.)

Incisions and Scars

Liposuction can be performed through small incisions, often less than one-fourth inch each. Usually, two incisions are needed to adequately treat each area. When possible, your incisions will be hidden in your pubic hair, inside your belly button, or in natural skin creases. Some areas, such as the hip, upper abdomen, and outer thigh, may require incisions that cannot be easily hidden. Because the scars are small, they usually are not noticeable once they mature.

What to Expect

When you arrive for surgery, your surgeon will mark the areas to be suctioned and may mark areas to avoid. This will be done with you standing, because the areas will shift when you recline. The marks help guide your surgeon during the operation. After you are sedated or asleep, your surgeon will make several tiny incisions around the areas to be treated. Using a long metal rod, about the diameter of a pencil, but much longer, your surgeon will inject tumescent fluid into your fat layer.

Following the infusion of tumescent fluid, your surgeon will use a *liposuction rod* to remove fat cells (figure 10-5). The rod has one or more holes at the end and will be attached to a suction machine or syringes, which produce a vacuum. Your plastic surgeon will then move the liposuction rod through your fat, systematically suctioning your deep fat.

Liposuction is performed under sedation or general anesthesia. Immediately following your procedure, your surgeon will place you in a liposuction garment (see next section). Unless you have large-volume liposuction, you will probably go home the same day.

Discomfort is variable but can be controlled with prescription pain medication. You will probably be able to return to work within one to two weeks and may resume exercise soon thereafter. But it is difficult to predict how quickly one will recover from this surgery.

Liposuction Garments

Liposuction garments are essential to achieving good results following surgery. They provide firm pressure and support to suctioned areas, facilitate skin retraction, and optimize your final contour. Most plastic surgeons will not perform liposuction unless a garment is available at the end of surgery. If you do not wear a properly fitted garment as instructed, you may have baggy, lumpy, irregular, and uneven results. Your surgeon will recommend that you wear your garment for

---

Tumescent Fluid

Tumescent *means overblown, turgid, ballooned, or inflated. Tumescent fluid is so named because its infusion makes the nearby fat temporarily stiff, which aids suctioning.*

Tumescent fluid contains saline, lidocaine (local anesthetic), and adrenaline. It reduces blood loss and improves the final result. Almost all plastic surgeons use tumescent fluid during liposuction. If your surgeon does not plan to do so, you may wish to seek another surgeon.

The Liposuction Rod

Liposuction rods, or cannulas, are long, thin, and available in a variety of diameters. The larger the rod, the more efficiently fat can be suctioned, and the quicker the procedure can be performed. Large rods are more likely to result in irregularities, lumpiness, uneven results, seromas, and fat emboli (see "complications"). Most plastic surgeons prefer medium and small rods, believing that the disadvantages of large rods outweigh their advantages.

Small rods: *2–3 millimeters in diameter*
Medium rods: *4–5 millimeters
    in diameter*
Large rods: *6–10 millimeters
    in diameter*

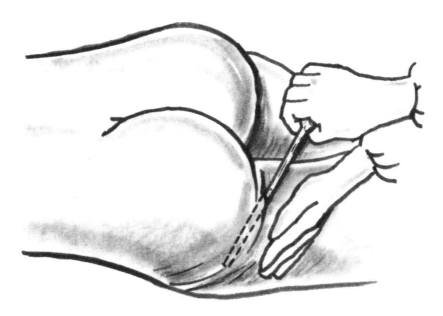

FIGURE 10-5: *Liposuction technique. The metal rod is moved methodically through your deep fat to evenly and effectively remove it.*

two to six weeks. Garments are designed to be worn continuously but may be removed daily for bathing. They are made of wash-and-wear material similar to spandex.

Your plastic surgeon may provide you with a garment or may ask you to order a garment by telephone prior to surgery. If you purchase it in advance, check the fit. Your garment should be very tight. If it seems to be a size too small, then it is probably the correct size. Garments cost $50 to $100 each, and you should purchase two if possible. You will be wearing them continuously for several weeks, and you will need to wear one while washing the other.

Liposuction garments are similar to girdles and vary in style according to areas suctioned. Garments must extend from below the lowest suctioned area to above the highest suctioned area. For liposuction of hips alone, your garment will resemble bicycle shorts. If you have liposuction of your hips, abdomen, and thighs, your garment will extend from knees to ribs.

To take a shower, remove your garment only if you are certain that you can put it back on afterward. This task will not be easy, because you will be swollen and sore, and the garment will be tight. If you anticipate

ANDIE, *a 27-year-old product design consultant, underwent a three-liter liposuction of her thighs and hips. She stopped taking pain medication in three days and was back to work within a week. Nina, Andie's 26-year-old friend, underwent a one-liter liposuction of her outer thighs and was incapacitated for two weeks. Recovery following liposuction simply varies from person to person.*

Vital Statistics

Anesthesia: *General or sedation.*

Location of operation: *Office or hospital.*

Length of surgery: *30 minutes to 5 hours, depending on the extent of fat to be removed.*

Length of stay: *Outpatient for small and medium volume; overnight for large volume.*

Discomfort: *Varies from mild to severe. Anticipate 2–14 days of prescription pain medication.*

Swelling: *Peaks within 3 days and dissipates over 2–8 weeks. As swelling resolves, it will settle to lower parts of your body. For example, following liposuction of your thighs, your knees and ankles will swell temporarily. Following liposuction of your abdomen, your genitalia will swell.*

Bruising: *Lasts for 2–10 days.*

Numbness and tingling: *May occur in suctioned areas and is due to damaged or irritated nerve endings. Sensation will return, and tingling will abate over 1–3 months. Regular self-massage of suctioned areas will expedite this process.*

Bandages: *Will be removed in 1–4 days.*

Stitches: *Will be removed in 5–10 days.*

Drains: *If drains are placed, they will be removed in 1–2 days.*

Support: *A liposuction garment must be worn continuously for 2–6 weeks.*

Presentable in a bathing suit: *You will be presentable once your bruising has resolved, your swelling has improved, and your plastic surgeon has allowed you to discontinue wearing your liposuction garment.*

Work: *Most can return to work in 5–14 days, if they have stopped taking prescription pain medication. If your job requires lifting, wait 2–3 weeks.*

Driving: *May be resumed after you have stopped taking prescription pain medication.*

Exercise: *May be resumed in 2–4 weeks. Exercise within 2 weeks of liposuction will increase swelling and postpone your final result.*

Final result: *Is seen after swelling subsides. Expect 4–8 weeks.*

difficulty replacing your garment, wear it in the shower and blow-dry it afterward. Garments may be machine laundered. If your garment is loose, the dryer will shrink it. If your garment is tight, allow it to air dry.

Volume of Fat Removed

Your plastic surgeon will know to stop suctioning based on the volume of fatty fluid suctioned and the appearance of the area. (Many surgeons keep a record of the volumes removed from each side of the body so that equal volumes are removed.) Before finishing an area, your surgeon should lightly suction the adjacent fat to blend the treated and untreated areas. This will create a smooth and natural result.

The typical volumes removed from each area are:

Neck	*25 to 100 ml*
Abdomen	*150 to 2,500 ml*
Hip (each)	*200 to 1,000 ml*
Outer thigh (each)	*300 to 2,000 ml*
Inner thigh (each)	*150 to 500 ml*
Front of thigh (each)	*200 to 1,200 ml*
Knee (each)	*50 to 100 ml*

For rough equivalents in U.S. liquid units of measure, 500 ml is about one pint, and 1,000 ml about one quart

The volumes shown include both fat and tumescent fluid.*

Large-Volume Liposuction

Women with marked fatty deposits may be candidates for removal of 10,000 ml or more. However, large-volume liposuction carries greater risk, and many plastic surgeons choose not to perform it. It involves longer operating times, more tumescent fluid infused, more fluid suctioned, and increased blood loss. (The more fluid that is put into and taken out of your body, the greater the stress to your body.) It also means a higher total dose of anesthetic.

Some plastic surgeons perform large-volume liposuction routinely and have found it to be safe. They closely monitor their patients during and after the procedure. The American Society of Plastic and Reconstructive Surgeons recommends that anyone undergoing more than five liters of liposuction stay one night in the hospital for observation.

If you and your surgeon are anticipating large-volume liposuction, be certain that you are in excellent health, your surgeon is experienced in this procedure, and you are monitored overnight in a hospital.

Most people seeking liposuction choose to have several areas suctioned at once. Commonly, 1,000 to 4,000 ml are removed during the procedure. Your surgeon may be able to predict the volume removed. More is not always better (see "Complications"). Do not request more liposuction than your surgeon recommends.

Complications

The media have deluged the public with liposuction horror stories. Unfortunately, most are true. Many, but not all, of the highly publicized complications occurred when liposuction was performed by unqualified doctors. When your operation is performed by a qualified plastic surgeon, you will increase your chances of an uneventful recovery.

Even in ideal circumstances, however, complications may occur. The risk of complications increases as the volume suctioned increases. In addition to specific complications mentioned here, refer to Chapter 1 for general complications that may follow any procedure.

Death

An estimated 25 people die each year in the United States from complications related to liposuction. Because the number of people having liposuction is approximately 250,000 per year, the risk of death is about 1 in 10,000. Some deaths have been due to puncture of internal organs with liposuction rods. This complication is preventable and is related to surgeon inexperience. Other complications may occur regardless of your surgeon's experience.

Fat Embolus

During liposuction, small fat globules may migrate into blood vessels and gather into a larger mass of fat. If it then travels into the lungs, it can interfere with respiration. Severe and potentially fatal problems may result. Fortunately, this occurs in less than 0.1 percent of liposuction patients. Even when it does occur, consequences are usually mild and improve with hospitalization and supplemental oxygen. Use of large-diameter liposuction rods may be linked with this problem.

When Can I Stop Worrying About Complications?

Most complications occur within a predictable period of time following surgery. If you do not develop them within the time periods noted, you can fairly conclude that you are probably free of these complications:

TIME AFTER SURGERY	POSSIBLE COMPLICA
3 days	*Heart failure*
3 days	*Bleeding*
2 weeks	*Fat embolus*
2 weeks	*Infection*
4 weeks	*DVT*
3 months	*Skin irregularities, dimples, puckers, di*
3 months	*Discoloration*

Deep Vein Thrombosis (DVT)

A deep vein thrombosis (DVT) is a blood clot in the deep veins of the thighs. It can travel through blood vessels and lodge in the lungs, leading to both potentially catastrophic breathing problems and debilitating leg problems. A blood clot can develop in your thigh even if you did not have liposuction in that particular area. DVT risk may be reduced if your surgeon applies leg compression devices during your operation.

Following surgery, a swollen or painful thigh may be a sign of a DVT. (However, everyone who has thigh liposuction gets swollen, painful thighs.) If one leg is more swollen than the other, an ultrasound scan can rule out a DVT. Be aware, however, that asymmetric swelling is common following liposuction, and does not necessarily mean a DVT is present. If you have any concerns about a possible DVT, call your surgeon at once. If a DVT is found, you will be admitted to the hospital for treatment and observation.

Heart Failure

During liposuction, you will be given lots of tumescent fluid and intravenous fluid. Most healthy people can tolerate this extra fluid load. However, if the load is extreme or if you have a weak heart, the fluid burden may cause your heart to fail. Normally this is easily treated with diuretics. But because heart failure can be fatal if severe or unrecognized, women with weak hearts should not have liposuction. For large-volume liposuction, which involves large fluid loads, even healthy people require close monitoring during and after surgery.

Bleeding

Blood loss depends on the amount of liposuction performed. About 75 ml of blood is lost with each 1,000 ml of fluid and fat suctioned. Average liposuction volumes of 1,000 to 4,000 ml result in 75 to 300 ml blood losses. Large-volume liposuction of 10,000 ml may remove 750 ml (1.5 pints) of blood. Most healthy people can handle this amount of blood loss with ease, but it may cause others to feel weak and anemic. Some patients will require transfusion. If your surgeon is planning large-volume liposuction, ask whether donating your own blood prior to surgery is an option.

Infection

Infection very rarely follows liposuction. If it does occur, it is usually mild and resolves with oral or intravenous antibiotics. An exceedingly rare, severe, and life-threatening infection, fasciitis, has been reported in a few cases. Fasciitis is so named because it spreads along a layer of tissue between fat and muscle, called *fascia*. Fasciitis is severe because of its rapid progression, its virulent strain of bacteria, or both. It is more common in diabetics because their immune systems are generally less robust. To treat fasciitis, antibiotics alone are inadequate; the infected skin and fat must be surgically removed. Eventually the open wounds are covered with skin grafts.

Irregularities, Dimples, Puckers, and Divots

One goal of liposuction is to create symmetric body contours with smooth and natural skin. Superficial liposuction, however, may lead to permanent skin irregularities, dimples, and depressions. Without enough fat to provide a cushion between skin and muscle, the body does not look natural. Fat injection can improve this problem.

Discoloration

Skin may become discolored in the area of liposuction. As swelling and bruising improve, blotchy patches may develop that are darker than your surrounding skin. During the healing phase, exposing your liposuctioned sites to unprotected sun will compound your risk of this unsightly complication. The overall risk is less than 5 percent of patients. Discoloration usually improves on its own within 3 to 12 months.

Telltale Signs

Irregularities, dimples, puckers, and divots, as described in the section on complications, may serve as telltale signs. However, many people who have not had liposuction may have these problems due to previous trauma or other surgeries. Therefore, they are not reliable telltale signs.

Cost

The average total fees for liposuction in the U.S. are shown in Table 10-1. These averages are rough guidelines. Nowhere in cosmetic surgery do costs vary more widely. See "Fees" in Chapter 1 for various fators that might affect your own cost.

Charges may be based on volume suctioned, specific areas suctioned, number of areas suctioned, or time spent suctioning. In general, the more

TABLE 10-1 *Average Cost of Liposuction*

	ONE AREA	THREE AREAS	FIVE AREAS
Surgeon's fee	$2,000	$5,000	$7,000
Anesthesiologist's fee	$ 500	$ 800	$1,000
Operating room (facility) fee	$ 700	$1,000	$1,200
Hospital fee for overnight stay	$ 0	$ 0	$ 500
Total	$3,200	$6,800	$9,700

Note: *Typically, each of the following counts as a single area: neck, abdomen, both hips, both flanks, both outer thighs, both inner thighs, or both knees. Many surgeons further subdivide areas, such as upper versus lower abdomen.*

you have suctioned, the more you will pay. And if you are considering ultrasonic or external ultrasound–assisted liposuction (discussed later in this chapter), then expect to pay $500 to $2,000 more.

Duration of Results

Fat cells are removed during liposuction. If your weight remains stable, your results following liposuction will be lasting. If you gain weight, your pattern of fat deposition cannot be predicted. Some women gain weight in previously suctioned areas. Although some fat cells were permanently removed, remaining fat cells may enlarge or multiply in response to weight gain.

Alternatively, future weight gain may appear in body sites not previously affected by weight gain. For example, after extensive liposuction of your abdomen, thighs, and hips, future weight gain may be deposited in your arms, neck, or calves. An altered pattern of weight gain is more common after numerous extensive liposuction procedures. In general, your pattern of future weight gain cannot be predicted. Controlling weight through diet and exercise is the best approach.

KALA, *a 28-year-old high school social studies teacher, had liposuction of her thighs and hips with good initial results. She gained weight afterward and returned one year later looking no different than she had looked before liposuction. During our discussion, she reached down, grabbed her hips, and said, "What's this? I thought you removed all this fat. I thought it was permanent." She requested touchup liposuction. I explained that her weight gain had caused fat to reaccumulate and that further liposuction was not warranted. I encouraged her instead to use diet and exercise to control her weight. Unfortunately, she left the office unhappy.*

Revision Liposuction

About 10–15 percent of those who have liposuction require revision. This is appropriate when asymmetric fat deposits persist after six months. Surgeons usually perform revision in the office with sedation, suctioning the larger area until it matches the smaller side.

Revision liposuction may be needed regardless of the experience of your surgeon. Partly this is because liposuction is performed when you are lying. If your surgeon could perform your liposuction with you in a standing position, many cases of revision might be avoided. Obviously, this is not possible. Therefore, your plastic surgeon cannot with certainty give you the result you expect.

If you do need revision, you should wait six months. Many surgeons will waive the surgeon's fee if performed within a certain period.

Realistic Expectations

Do not expect all fat to be removed from treated areas. This would look unnatural, and it is impossible, anyway. The right amount of fat to remove is that which brings your contour into harmony with the rest of your body. If your silhouette looks like a cello, expect that your convex and concave curves will be smoothed, as noted with the dotted line (fig. 10-3 a). You will likely discover that your measurements have improved, and you may wear smaller clothing by one or more sizes. Weight is sometimes reduced—but not always.

Liposuction Techniques

The popularity of liposuction has led to modifications of the traditional technique with the goals of better results and fewer complications. Two newer techniques incorporate ultrasound waves into liposuction treatments. But do they really offer any advantages?

Terminology

Some plastic surgeons use alternative terms for liposuction, such as lipoplasty, liposculpture, or lipectomy. They are not offering a new or better technique, but may be trying to convince you they are.

Traditional Liposuction

Traditional liposuction began in the 1970s. It remains the most common technique for cosmetic fat removal. (The technique for liposuction described earlier in this chapter is for traditional liposuction.)

Advantages

Traditional liposuction has been practiced for nearly 30 years, and it yields consistent and satisfying results when performed by experienced plastic surgeons. No long-term negative consequences have been identified. Nearly all plastic surgeons who perform liposuction have experience with this technique. More experience translates into better results. Because high-tech equipment is not needed, it often costs less than newer techniques.

What's in a Name?

Traditional liposuction *may also be called:* liposuction, standard liposuction, tumescent liposuction, wet liposuction, super-wet liposuction, lipoplasty, traditional lipoplasty, standard lipoplasty, tumescent lipoplasty, liposculpture, traditional liposculpture, standard liposculpture, tumescent liposculpture, suction lipectomy, suction assisted lipectomy (SAL), tumescent suction assisted lipectomy, and other names.

Ultrasonic liposuction (UL) *may also be called:* ultrasound assisted liposuction (UAL), standard ultrasonic liposuction, ultrasonic lipoplasty, ultrasound assisted lipoplasty, ultrasonic liposculpture, ultrasound assisted liposculpture, ultrasonic lipectomy, ultrasonic suction lipectomy, ultrasound assisted suction lipectomy, and other names.

External ultrasound–assisted liposuction (EUAL) *may also be called:* external ultrasound–assisted lipoplasty, external ultrasound–assisted liposculpture, external ultrasound–assisted lipectomy, and other names.

DISADVANTAGES

Traditional liposuction may remove more blood than techniques that employ ultrasonic energy. This matters most in large-volume liposuction, where blood loss can be substantial.

Ultrasonic Liposuction

Ultrasonic liposuction (UL) was developed in Europe in the 1980s and was first used in the United States in the early 1990s. It became widely available in the United States in 1995. Ultrasonic liposuction combines the application of high-frequency sound waves with gentle suctioning.

First, tumescent fluid is instilled, as in traditional liposuction. Second, your surgeon inserts a rod capable of emitting ultrasonic waves into your fat. The waves liquefy the nearby fat. Liquefied fat is then easily removed by gentle suctioning.

ADVANTAGES

Compared to traditional liposuction, UL may be less traumatic to fibrous tissue, blood vessels, and remaining fat. Less suction power is needed. This may translate into less pain, swelling, blood loss, and bruising, and speedier recovery. Skin retraction may be superior. Further clinical studies are needed to prove that these presumed advantages are real.

Ultrasonic liposuction seems most beneficial in two settings. In large-volume liposuction, the ultrasonic technique may result in less blood loss. Ultrasonic liposuction may also offer an advantage in revision liposuction because of its ability to soften fat before suctioning. (Following liposuction, any fat left behind is tougher and more difficult to suction.)

DISADVANTAGES

Because the equipment needed is expensive, UL may not be available everywhere. Many surgeons charge approximately $500 more per site for UL. The incisions are slightly larger. You may sustain a skin burn near a treated area, although burns are rare and easily prevented through proper technique. Fluid collections, called seromas, are more common following UL than traditional liposuction. (Seroma incidence may be reduced by drain placement at the time of surgery. The drain can then be removed in the office a few days later.) Following UL, patients are more likely to develop painful tingling of their skin, which may persist for several months. Ultrasonic liposuction takes longer, which may translate into higher cost and surgical risks. It is not suited for knees, neck, and calves, because of characteristics of the liposuction rod. Finally, the long-term effects of ultrasonic energy, as delivered through liposuction, are not known.

External Ultrasound–Assisted Liposuction (EUAL)

External ultrasound–assisted liposuction (EUAL) became widely available in 1997. In UL, ultrasonic waves are delivered through a rod that is inserted into fat. Because the rod is placed beneath the skin, ultrasonic energy can be delivered directly to fat. In EUAL, ultrasonic energy is delivered to skin overlying the fat. Then liposuction is performed.

ADVANTAGES

When compared to traditional liposuction, EUAL, like UL, may offer the advantages of less blood loss, less swelling, less discomfort, and faster recovery. When compared to UL, EUAL may also offer decreased risks of seromas, burns, and painful postoperative tingling.

DISADVANTAGES

None of the supposed advantages have been proved, and many plastic surgeons remain skeptical. EUAL is more expensive and time-consuming than traditional liposuction. Like UL, the long-term effects of ultrasonic energy, as delivered during the procedure, are not known.

Assessing the Three Techniques

The claims of smoother results and shorter recoveries with ultrasonic techniques have not been proved. Also, long-term effects of ultrasonic energy on the human body, as applied through liposuction, are not yet known.

Because of its relative infancy, large studies on EUAL are lacking. More time and information are needed. Long-term results and safety will not be known for decades.

Many plastic surgeons prefer ultrasonic liposuction because they have noted advantages without increased complications. Other plastic surgeons prefer traditional liposuction to ultrasonic liposuction because they find that the potential disadvantages outweigh the presumed advantages. Some plastic surgeons have tried ultrasonic liposuction but have returned to traditional liposuction after finding no clear benefit. Clearly, we have not reached a consensus on which technique is superior.

Satisfaction

Satisfaction following liposuction is closely tied to expectations. If you expect significant weight reduction or improvement in cellulite following liposuction, you will be disappointed. If you expect a more harmonious body contour and understand the limitations, you probably will be pleased.

Concluding Thoughts

Several liposuction techniques exist to help you achieve your desired results. Comparison studies show no significant difference in final results. Among plastic surgeons, there is no consensus regarding the optimal technique. When you seek liposuction, follow the advice of your plastic surgeon, who will recommend the technique that yields the best results in his or her hands.

Liposuction reduces specific areas of fat which are otherwise resistant to diet and exercise. It involves permanent removal of fat cells from the body. Provided there is no weight gain, results are lasting. For these reasons, liposuction has become the most popular procedure in cosmetic surgery.

Questions to Ask Your Plastic Surgeon

What size liposuction rods do you use?

Do you use tumescent fluid?

What is your revision rate?

What is your revision policy?

Which liposuction technique do you recommend and why?

Will my procedure be performed in a hospital?

Tips and Traps

Wait until your body weight has been stable for at least six months before seeking liposuction.

Do not expect liposuction to improve your cellulite. It may actually worsen it.

Maintain stable weight following liposuction for the best results.

You cannot predict where you will gain weight following liposuction. You may regain weight in the area of liposuction, or you may develop fat deposits in other places.

If you seek large volume liposuction, find a surgeon who is experienced and anticipate an overnight hospital stay.

Consider a lift rather than liposuction if you have significantly loose skin.

For the sake of good body contour, surgeons sometimes wisely recommend liposuction of adjacent areas, such as hips or thighs.

Avoid liposuction of buttock creases and calves unless your surgeon is highly experienced in liposuction of these areas.

Plastic surgeons are divided over which liposuction technique is best.

11

Smoothing Your Wrinkles with Simple Solutions

Skin Care, Micro Peels, Superficial Peels, Wrinkle Fillers, and Botox

Rough, lifeless, blotchy, and wrinkled skin can be aggravating. Relatively simple options are available to improve it. The solutions aim to brighten the complexion, smooth the skin, revitalize the face, equalize the color, and improve fine wrinkles—all while allowing immediate recovery, imposing little risk, and being relatively inexpensive.

Anything that sounds too good to be true probably is. Such is the case with simple solutions for wrinkles. Each approach has limitations—and requires multiple treatments.

All simple solutions need to be performed regularly for best results. Skin care, for example, should be performed twice a day at home. Micro peels should be performed twice a month for three months, then maintained quarterly. Filler injections and Botox also require regular treatments.

No Such Thing as a Healthy Tan

Before considering any skin problem or treatment, it is critical that you first understand the damaging effects of ultraviolet light. Ultraviolet light (from the sun or tanning beds) accelerates and compounds the aging process. The effects of ultraviolet light are cumulative and delayed. If you have significant sun exposure during your teens, you may not see sun

HELEN, *a 43-year-old homemaker, won a recipe contest that was sponsored by a local television show. She was both elated and panicked when she was invited to appear on the program. She wanted to look her best, but with just two weeks to prepare, her options were limited. Two micropeels and Botox injections of her forehead, frown lines, and crow's feet helped her to feel her best the day the show was filmed.*

damage for decades. But by that time, avoiding the sun will not prevent accelerated aging. The greater your lifetime total ultraviolet light exposure, the greater the damage to your skin. The term "photoaging" is often used to describe the changes that occur to sun-damaged skin over time.

Most important, exposure to ultraviolet light increases your chance of developing skin cancer. The greater your lifetime exposure, the greater your risk. Melanoma, a particularly aggressive type of skin cancer, may be fatal even when diagnosed and treated early. Clearly, there are many reasons to protect yourself from the damaging effects of the sun.

Identify Your Skin Problems

To begin your quest for youthful skin, first take inventory of your specific problems. This will help you select the treatment(s) most appropriate for you.

Loss of Skin Vitality

Skin vitality is a feature that is difficult to quantify and describe. It is related to skin color and brightness— irrespective of tone, wrinkles, or texture. Skin with vitality appears young, healthy, energetic, and colorful. Skin with loss of vitality appears old, lifeless, tired, and pale.

Discolorations

Discolorations are discolored patches of skin that are usually darker than surrounding skin. Some color irregularities are superficial and some are deep. Their depth determines which treatment is most appropriate. Superficial discoloration such as age spots are improved with many treatments. (Deep discoloration, such as deep melasma, are further described in Chapter 13.)

MEG, *a 39-year-old sun worshipper, lived in the Sun Belt and prided herself on her deep tan. When work and weather kept her from the sun, she went to tanning booths. By the age of 30, her skin looked like that of a 40-year-old. By the age of 35, her skin looked like that of a 50-year-old. She finally realized that her sun exposure must stop. She was horrified, however, to see that her accelerated aging did not then stop. By the age of 39, she had the skin of a 60-year-old. Skin does not forget its previous sun exposure, and the full effects of sun damage may be delayed by years.*

Sources of Ultraviolet Light

Sun damages your skin through ultraviolet A (UVA) light. Protection against ultraviolet light through use of sunscreens will reduce its negative effect. Tanning beds emit ultraviolet B (UVB) light, which may be more damaging than natural UVA light. Most sunscreens only protect against UVA light. If you have worn sunscreen into tanning beds, you have likely received no protection from UVB light. Both UVA and UVB light are harmful to your skin and promote aging. There is no such thing as a healthy tan.

Skin Roughness

Roughness relates to skin texture. In youth, skin is smooth, but with age, it becomes more rough and irregular.

Large Pores

Although some women are burdened with large pores in youth, many do not develop this problem until later in life. Large pores are visible and unattractive. Small pores are considered more desirable.

Wrinkles

All wrinkles are not treated equally. Treatment depends on the cause of the wrinkle . Each cause generates a specific type of wrinkle.

CREPE-PAPER WRINKLES FROM PHOTOAGED SKIN

Crepe-paper wrinkles are fine wrinkles that occur on the cheeks, where sun exposure is high and the skin is relatively thin and sensitive to its effects.

DYNAMIC WRINKLES FROM FACIAL MUSCLES

The most troublesome and abundant facial wrinkles are *dynamic wrinkles*, also called "smile lines" and "frown lines." They are the result of facial expressions we make hundreds of thousands of times over a lifetime. When we smile, laugh, frown, or brood, the skin of our faces is repeatedly moved. Each time the skin moves, it creases and eventually forms wrinkles.

Dynamic wrinkles may occur anywhere we have facial muscles, but they are worst in a few areas. The forehead has horizontal wrinkles (due to raising the eyebrows) and vertical wrinkles between the brows (due to scowling). Crow's feet develop around the eyes from smiling and squinting. Vertical wrinkles develop around the lips due to pursing them (fig. 11-1).

Dynamic wrinkles are depressions or narrow troughs within the skin. Because they are lower than the skin on either side, light casts shadows into them. The deeper the wrinkle, the greater the shadow, and the more it is visible.

SKIN FOLD WRINKLES FROM DROOPING CHEEKS

Skin fold wrinkles may occur as your cheeks begin to sag. Skin folds, called nasolabial folds, can develop around your nose and mouth (fig. 11-2). As your skin folds develop, wrinkles will accompany them.

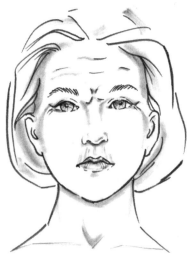

FIGURE 11-1: *Wrinkles due to facial expressions. Note the forehead horizontal wrinkles, scowl lines between the eyebrows, crow's feet, and vertical lip wrinkles.*

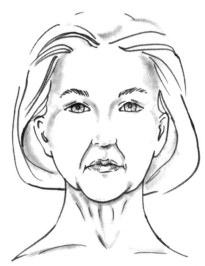

FIGURE 11-2: *Wrinkles due to skin folds. The heavy nasolabial folds are caused by the sagging cheeks; the wrinkle accompanies the folds.*

Loss of Skin Tone

Skin tone may be poor due to genetics and is worsened with aging and sun exposure. Loss of skin tone is evident by loose, droopy cheeks.

Overview of Skin Treatments

Skin care and micro peels renew vitality by expediting skin turnover and bringing younger, healthier skin to the surface. Wrinkle fillers, such as collagen, do not affect quality or tone of skin, but camouflage dynamic wrinkles by raising them to the height of surrounding skin. Botox works on dynamic wrinkles by weakening the responsible muscles. The table titled "Treatment Options" summarizes these simple solutions, which will be discussed in this chapter. For comparison, the table also shows more serious solutions; see Chapter 12 for details.

Regarding skin fold wrinkles, a face-lift is usually the best treatment (see Chapter 2). It can tighten facial skin, improve heavy skin folds, and soften the associated wrinkles. Profound loss of skin tone is also best treated with

TABLE 11-1 *Treatment Options*

| | | | SIMPLE SOLUTIONS | | SERIOUS SOLUTIONS | | | | |
	FILLERS	BOTOX	SKIN CARE	MICRO AND SUPERFICIAL PEEL	MEDIUM PEEL	LASER: ERBIUM	DERM-ABRASION	LASER: CO₂	DEEP PEEL
Large pore size			++	+++	++				
Loss of vitality			++	+++	++	+			
Rough skin			++	+++	+++	+++	+++	+++	+++
Fine wrinkles			+	+	++	+++	+++	+++	+++
Discoloration			+	+	++	++	++	++	+++
Loss of skin tone					+	++	+	++	++
Acne scars						++	++	++	+
Dynamic wrinkles	+	+++				+	++	++	+++
Recovery (days)	0	0	0	0	4–7	4–7	7–10	10–14	10–14

face-lift. Deep chemical peels, laser, and dermabrasion (Chapter 12) can promote a more modest degree of skin tightening.

Skin Care

Your skin is composed of damaged superficial cells and healthier deep cells. Every day, superficial cells die, shed, and are replaced by younger cells. This process becomes disorganized and inefficient as you age. The older you are, the longer it may take to shed unhealthy cells, leaving you with a lifeless complexion.

Skin care and micro chemical peels cause controlled injury to your damaged superficial cells, resulting in their uniform destruction and shedding. This allows the healthier deep cells to surface while they are still young and fresh. Skin turnover is organized, expedited, and helps you reclaim the skin of your youth.

The goal of skin care is to decrease roughness, brighten your complexion, minimize pore size, reduce blotches, and provide a healthier overall appearance. Some women also benefit through subtle improvement of fine wrinkles.

Improvement in dynamic wrinkles, however, will not occur. The changes seen with skin care occur subtly over six to twelve months.

Micro peels and superficial peels (covered later in this chapter) are an important and effective adjunct to a comprehensive skin care program.

Balanced Skin Care Programs

A balanced skin care program is set up and monitored by a nurse or skin care technician who will evaluate your skin and outline a program suited to your needs. A comprehensive skin care program will be geared toward four goals: exfoliation, stimulation, medication, and protection. These goals will be achieved through daily or twice-daily home application of cleansers, alpha hydroxy acids, retin-A, bleaching agents, sunscreen, and moisturizers. The frequency of application and concentration of these agents can be increased as your skin becomes accustomed to them. If your skin reacts with redness or rash, your program will be tailored appropriately.

Skin Care Products

MILD CLEANSERS

You will begin skin care each day with a mild cleanser, which lifts off dead superficial skin cells. This process of exfoliation facilitates penetration of stimulants such as alpha hydroxy acid and retin-A.

ALPHA HYDROXY ACIDS

Alpha hydroxy acids (AHAs) are naturally occurring acids that stimulate growth and turnover of skin cells. Their sources are:

AHA	*Source*
Glycolic acid	*Sugar cane*
Citric acid	*Oranges and grapefruits*
Malic acid	*Apples*
Lactic acid	*Milk*

The most commonly used AHA is glycolic acid. It is available in concentrations of 4–15 percent for home use. Depending on your skin sensitivity, you may be started at a low or medium concentration until you demonstrate tolerance. The acids work by thickening the deep layers of your skin, resulting

Principles Behind Skin Care Products

Exfoliation: *Cleansers remove dead skin cells so that other agents can penetrate.*

Stimulation: AHAs *and retin-A enhance new skin growth and turnover.*

Medication: *Bleaching agents treat or prevent discoloration for those at risk.*

Protection: *Moisturizers and sunscreen protect your skin from further damage.*

in improved skin texture, complexion, smoothness, and appearance. The effects of AHA are enhanced by concurrent use of retin-A.

(Beta hydroxy acids, or BHAs, such as salicylic acid, may also be incorporated into skin care. These acids may offer even greater improvement than AHAs for some people.)

RETIN-A

Retin-A is short for *retinoic acid,* also called "tretinoin." Retin-A stimulates circulation to your skin and facilitates skin cell growth and turnover. It thickens the deep layers of your skin, leading to a brighter, healthier complexion with smoother texture. Retin-A will help reduce fine wrinkles, but will not affect dynamic wrinkles or skin-fold wrinkles.

When retin-A was initially introduced in the 1970s, the mass media reported that it offered significant improvement in wrinkles. Most physicians who prescribed retin-A were careful to explain that it would not affect dynamic wrinkles. Because of the overwhelming impact of the media, most consumers expected retin-A to eliminate all wrinkles and were greatly disappointed when it did not. This lead to widespread disappointment in the product. This is unfortunate because the other improvements seen with retin-A are real.

One genuine disadvantage of retin-A is that it may cause skin irritation even in low concentrations. You may develop a temporary rash or experience a transient burning sensation while using it. (In order to help you develop tolerance to retin-A, you may be asked to temporarily decrease the amount of retin-A you apply, decrease the frequency of application, increase moisturizer use, or apply steroid cream. You will slowly be graduated to medium or strong concentrations of retin-A to achieve the maximum benefit.) Another disadvantage of retin-A is that it may worsen facial spider veins by stimulating blood flow. (If you have problematic spider veins, you may choose to have them treated with laser before you start retin-A.) Finally, retin-A causes dry skin. Moisturizers alone may overcome this. If not, you may switch from retin-A to Renova. Renova is similar but has less drying effect. Many doctors and skin care specialists believe retin-A is more effective and will ask you to continue retin-A if possible. Despite the problems retin-A may cause, its effect on skin, when used consistently, can be dramatic.

BLEACHING AGENTS

Bleaching agents, such as hydroquinone, can be helpful in the prevention and treatment of blotchy, discolored skin. Bleaching agents do not actually bleach skin; rather they suppress the activity of pigment-producing cells. If your skin is not blotchy or discolored, you will not need bleaching agents as part of your skin care program. If you plan to pursue chemical peel or laser resurfacing, you may temporarily require bleaching agents for prevention of dark discoloration.

MOISTURIZERS

Moisturizers will keep your skin healthy and soft while your superficial, unhealthy skin layers are shed. They will also help you tolerate the drying effects of retin-A.

SUNSCREEN

Sunscreen is essential to the success of a balanced skin care program for two reasons. Your skin care program should heighten your awareness of the damaging effects of the sun and should make you eager to protect yourself from further damage. Also, an effective skin care program will actually increase your skin's sensitivity to sun and make you more likely to sustain a burn than if you were not using skin care products.

Beware Costly and Ineffective Products

Skin care products available through department stores, beauty salons, and drug stores may claim they are effective and boast "20% glycolic acid" or higher. Yet these products may offer little improvement when compared to skin care products obtained through your plastic surgeon. The effect of glycolic acid, and all AHAS, depends on pH (acidity). Products obtained through a physician will have the appropriate pH for optimal results.

pH 1–2	*Strong acid—the typical pH of effective skin care products obtained from your plastic surgeon*
pH 3–4	*Medium acid*
pH 5–6	*Weak acid*
pH 7	*No acid (neutral)—the typical pH of skin care products obtained outside of a doctor's office*

A preparation of glycolic acid with a neutral pH will be ineffective compared to your plastic surgeon's glycolic acid with an acidic pH, regardless of concentration. The products available in stores are safe; however, they also have little effect on your skin.

Physician Supervised Skin Care Programs

"Physician supervised" means that a physician has ensured that the technician, nurse, or aesthetician has been properly trained to administer skin care programs and perform safe and effective micro peels. It does not mean that the physician will be present at the time of your skin care evaluation or peel. Nor does it mean that you will necessarily meet the physician.

Physician supervised skin care programs are able to obtain and distribute the most highly effective skin care products. The more effective a skin care product, the greater is its potential to cause skin irritation and increased sensitivity to the sun. Thus, these products must be administered by a trained medical professional. Your day spa or department store may insist that their products are effective, but be suspicious unless their programs are physician supervised. Few are.

Recovery

Skin care requires no recovery time. You may apply makeup immediately following application of your skin care products.

Cost

The program is affordable with an average monthly cost of $30 to $50.

Duration of Results

Skin care will maintain your skin vitality and smoothness as long as you use the products regularly. If you stop using them, expect your skin to return to baseline within three to six months.

Satisfaction

Because physician supervised skin care programs are safe, effective, and affordable, satisfaction is immense. The few who are disappointed are those who fail to use the products consistently and those who expect too much.

Micro Peels and Superficial Peels

Micro Peels

Micro peels are an important adjunct to any skin care program. Most people who pursue skin care programs choose to boost their skin care results with concomitant micro peels.

> **BRANDY**, *a 43-year-old department store salesperson, was pleased with her skin care program, but desired more improvement. She had micro peels every two weeks for three months and developed a brighter, healthier complexion. Skin care and bimonthly micro peels then maintained this fresh appearance.*

Micro peels, like other chemical peels, apply a chemical irritant to the skin. They are performed in a doctor's office by a trained skin care technician or nurse and require about 30 minutes. First, dead skin cells are gently removed through a painless technique called derma planing, which is similar to shaving. Then a glycolic acid solution, usually between 30 and 50 percent, is applied. You may experience mild, temporary burning and itching. Stimulants such as dry ice may then be applied, followed by moisturizing cream. Immediately following your micro peel, you can apply makeup and return to your usual activities. Most will have no outward evidence of the peel, but those with fair skin may have a red complexion for a day.

Following each peel, your dead superficial skin cells will invisibly shed. You will see the biggest effect two weeks later. Six peels are usually required at two-week intervals to achieve peak results. Thereafter, you may maintain that level with micro peels every two to three months. Micro peels work best when combined with a skin care program.

Advantages

Micro peels offer significant advantage over skin care products alone, because they are more potent, yet recovery is immediate. A micro peel will improve your skin texture, color, and overall appearance as well as decrease the apparent size of your pores. Many experience improvement in the superficial, crepe-paper wrinkles.

Disadvantages

As long as your expectations are realistic, disadvantages are few. A micro peel will not improve dynamic wrinkles, skin fold wrinkles, or skin tone.

If you have thin, sensitive skin, you may have redness for one or two days following your micro peel. If this occurs, a lower concentration of solution will be used for subsequent peels.

Superficial Peels

Superficial peels employ chemicals that are slightly stronger than those used for micro peels. Because of this, superficial peels are more effective in improving skin texture, vitality, and freshness. However, they result in visible flaking, which gives the appearance of extremely dry skin. Flaking begins one day after the peel and ends one to three days later. Hence, superficial peels are often called weekend peels. You may engage in your normal activities immediately following your superficial peel. But, if you have an important event planned, you will not want to have a superficial peel within four days of that event.

To achieve optimal results, have your superficial peel repeated monthly for six months. Thereafter, additional peels every two or three months will maintain your result. As with all peels, adherence to a physician-supervised skin care program will enhance your results and make them more lasting.

Advantages

As with micro peels, a nurse or trained skin care technician may perform a superficial peel. Therefore, the price is lower than medium peels, which are performed by physicians.

Disadvantages

Because monthly treatments are recommended to achieve optimal results, this means a few days of visible flaking each month for half a year. Not everyone's schedule can tolerate this.

Is the Skin Care Professional Qualified?

A skin care technician or nurse should perform your micro peel or superficial peel. If you receive your peel in the office of a plastic surgeon, you can be confident that the person performing it is appropriately trained. If you are in a nonmedical setting, then one of two things may occur:

- *The solutions used may be ineffective.*
- *The solutions may be effective and obtained as contraband.*

In the former case, no harm done— but no improvement either. In the latter case, you may be at risk for serious complications, because the person applying the products may not be properly trained or physician supervised.

Chemicals and Safety Valves

A number of different chemicals may be used to achieve a superficial peel. These include glycolic acid, resorcinol, salicylic acid, and others. Multiple reputable brand names exist, and new superficial peeling agents are added to the market regularly. Brands include Blue Peel, Jessner's Solution, and Micro Peel Plus.

Some peels have built-in safety valves to prevent the technician from allowing the chemical agent to overpenetrate. For example, one safety valve involves painting your skin with blue dye beforehand. Then the technician who performs your peel knows to stop when the blue color disappears. Because any peeling agent can cause a burn with subsequent scarring, a physician should supervise the person performing your superficial peel.

Cost

Micro peels cost $60 to $80 per peel. The average cost of a superficial peel is $80 to $120 per peel.

Duration of Results

Micro peels and superficial peels both require maintenance. Following your first six peels, you must continue using skin care products regularly at home and have maintenance peels every two or three months. If you cannot follow this regime, expect your skin to return to baseline within six months.

Satisfaction

Because micro peels and superficial peels are safe, effective, and affordable, satisfaction is immense. The few who are disappointed either fail to sustain their results through maintenance peels or expect too much.

Wrinkle Fillers

Wrinkles are visible because they are lower or deeper than surrounding skin. Light casts shadows into them, making them visible. When you see wrinkles, you are actually looking at the shadow, not the wrinkle. If wrinkles can be brought to the same level as surrounding skin, their visibility will diminish because the accompanying shadows will vanish. This can be accomplished by either lowering the surrounding skin or raising each wrinkle. Chemical peel, dermabrasion, and laser aim to lower the surrounding skin. Fillers aim to raise the wrinkle.

A colleague tells of a patient, a 67-year-old retired schoolteacher who complained to her hair stylist about her wrinkles. Before her hair was dry, another woman appeared, touting the miracles of chemical peels. Following her hair appointment, she stayed for a peel. It burned intensely, but she assumed that the woman performing her peel was qualified. It took her three weeks to heal, and she was left with permanent scars on her neck. She has since undergone corrective surgery but has not regained a natural appearance. Had she the opportunity to turn back the clock, she would have gladly kept her wrinkles.

Options for Wrinkle Fillers

Bovine collagen *is extracted from cow skin, then purified, sterilized, and processed into liquid form.*

Autologen *is collagen from your own skin, harvested during a previous operation and processed into liquid form.*

Isolagen *is collagen from your own skin, cloned in a laboratory and processed into liquid form.*

Dermalogen *is collagen from human cadaver skin that has been sterilized, purified, and processed into liquid form.*

Fat *is harvested from your own body through liposuction, then filtered and reinjected.*

Fillers are agents such as collagen or fat. Using fine needles, your plastic surgeon can inject fillers into your skin under each wrinkle. The filler pushes the depressed wrinkle outward and makes it less visible.

Collagen and Related Substances

Collagen is the protein matrix of the skin and is sometimes called the "meat" of the skin. It may be obtained from cow skin, cadaver skin, or your own skin. It is refined, sterilized, and processed so that it may be used safely. The improvement seen after collagen injection is not usually permanent. As a rule, implant materials such as collagen last longest if they are injected into skin, which is composed of collagen, rather than into fat beneath the skin. Because skin is more sensitive than fat, collagen injections are more painful than injections under the skin, such as Botox (see later in this chapter).

Types of Fillers

Collagen is prepared in thick liquid form suitable for injection through a small needle. So far, four types of collagen are used for cosmetic injection: bovine collagen, Autologen, Isolagen, and Dermalogen.

Bovine Collagen

Bovine collagen is derived from cow skin and has been the mainstay of collagen therapy for decades. Bovine collagen injections have a number of drawbacks such as short-lived duration, allergic reactions, and association with connective tissue disorders.

Bovine collagen is absorbed over weeks to months, thereby offering only temporary help. If you pursue bovine collagen injections, plan to receive injections every six weeks to three months. (Occasionally, bovine collagen injections may last six months.) Because the effect is transient, your surgeon will probably over-fill your wrinkles. They may temporarily look too full, but will last longer.

Some people are allergic to bovine collagen. To determine if you are allergic, you must undergo two skin tests in which a small amount of bovine collagen is injected into your forearm. If you do not develop redness by the end of one month, then you may safely receive collagen injections. Allergy occurs in fewer than 5 percent of the population.

Some doctors believe that about 1 in 10,000 who have bovine collagen injections may be predisposed to developing connective tissue disorders, such as lupus or arthritis. Other doctors feel that medical evidence to support this is lacking. There is no way to predict who, if anyone, is at risk. If such a disease develops, it may persist long after you have stopped receiving bovine collagen injections.

Collagen injections can be performed in the office and require less than 15 minutes. Most women can return to work or normal activities immediately, but mild redness, irritation, and swelling may last a few days.

AUTOLOGEN

Autologen is processed skin, derived from your own excess skin. Excess skin may be obtained as a result of operations such as tummy tuck, face-lift, or breast lift. Normally, excess skin is discarded following such operations. Your skin will instead be sent to a commercial laboratory that extracts collagen and prepares it for reinjection. One month later, your collagen is sent back to your surgeon. The amount of collagen yielded depends on the amount of skin removed. About one ml of liquid collagen can be extracted from three square inches of skin. Expect to obtain about four ml from tummy tuck skin, which is enough to fill several facial wrinkles three to five times.

Your plastic surgeon will inject about one ml per visit. Injections may be performed at one to three month intervals, and a total of three injections are typically performed. Your processed liquid collagen can be stored for five years if you do not need it all at once.

Your own collagen is unlikely to trigger an allergic reaction, and connective tissue diseases have not been associated with it. Although Autologen injections appear to last longer than bovine collagen injections, duration is variable. Some doctors may claim that the effect is permanent. If your doctor says this, be skeptical. This has not been proved.

The drawback, of course, is that you must first have surgery in which excess skin is removed. If you seek such an operation, then this may not be a drawback.

ISOLAGEN

Isolagen is a relatively new technology. Isolagen is cloned (cultured is actually the correct term) in a laboratory from a small sample of your skin. First, your plastic surgeon removes a piece of skin the size of a pencil eraser from behind your ear and sends it to the Isolagen lab in New Jersey. Within a few weeks, the lab will send back your cloned collagen-making cells.

Isolagen is composed of live cells that make collagen, called *fibroblasts*, rather than collagen itself. These cells are alive and must be injected the day they reach your surgeon; otherwise, they will be useless.

A minimum of three injections of one ml each are recommended at two week intervals. The first injection will improve your wrinkles by about 15 percent, the second injection by 35 percent, and the third injection by 70 percent. Because live cells are injected, improvement may continue for several months after the last injection.

Isolagen, unlike bovine collagen, theoretically does not need maintenance injections. Presumably, the benefit gained will eventually dissipate, and you will need another series of injections. Whether your next set of injections will be within months or years of your first is not known.

Because Isolagen is derived from your own skin, allergic reactions or development of connective tissue disorders are rare. Because actual live cells are injected, the effect of Isolagen may last years, according to the manufacturer. Some recipients may have permanent improvement, but this has not been proved. Isolagen is suited for wrinkles of the cheeks and lips, but not for lip augmentation, crow's feet, or forehead wrinkles.

Isolagen became available widely only in 1998. Your physician may not be familiar with it. Keep in mind, as you pursue this or any other new technology, that until it has been used on a large number of patients over decades, long-term results and potential problems will not be known.

DERMALOGEN

Dermalogen is another relatively new option in collagen-related materials. It is obtained from deceased human donors (see the sidebar in Chapter 6 titled "Tissues from Deceased Donors"). It is processed in liquid form for injection into lips or wrinkles. It may last longer than bovine collagen and minimizes allergic reactions and connective tissue disorders. Unlike Isolagen or Autologen, it neither requires skin removal nor a waiting period. Transmission of infection from the human donor is a theoretical risk, but because Dermalogen is sterilized and processed, it has not occurred.

Two or three injections are recommended at one to two month intervals to achieve best results. Then the benefit is expected to dissipate over months or years, at which time a new series of injections will be needed.

Cost

Bovine collagen injection costs $500 to $800 per visit. This includes the surgeon's fee and the cost of collagen, which is $150 to $200 per ml from the manufacturer. Typically, one ml is injected during each visit, which is enough to fill several wrinkles.

Autologen is slightly more expensive than bovine collagen. The average cost of preparing Autologen is $550 for the first three ml and $800 total if more than three ml are prepared. Your surgeon will charge an additional $350 to $500 per ml for each injection, and usually three injections are performed.

The cost of Isolagen is $500 for each one ml preparation. Your surgeon will charge an additional $750 to $1000 to perform each injection. If you have the recommended three injections, your total cost will be about $4,000.

Cost of Dermalogen is $150 per ml and your surgeon's fee for injection will average $500 to $750 per session.

Fat Injection

Fat needs little introduction, other than to say that most people have adequate stores for harvest. Fat can be harvested through liposuction and reinjected. Fat injection, like bovine collagen injection, has a reputation for providing only temporary augmentation. The duration depends on the tissue into which the fat is injected and the technique used by your plastic surgeon.

The tissue into which fat is injected plays the most important role. Because fat injections fare best when injected into fat, and because wrinkles are within the skin, many plastic surgeons think that fat injection for wrinkles is doomed to failure. Fat injected into skin will not last, and fat injected into fat will not improve wrinkles.

The other critical factor in determining survival of your fat injection is the technique for harvesting, filtering, preparing, and reinjecting. Experienced plastic surgeons have refined their technique and can create smooth, symmetric, lasting results when injecting fat into fat. Inexperienced surgeons can create irregularities, lumps, and pits that are difficult to correct.

Even in the best of circumstances, your injected fat is expected to shrink by 30 to 50 percent over the first few months. For this reason, many plastic surgeons recommend "over-injection" by about 50 percent. Initially the area treated may appear unnaturally full, but the augmentation will last longer and more closely approach your desired result.

Anticipate one to three injection sessions, perhaps many more, before your desired result is achieved. Fat injection can be performed in the office with local anesthesia. Only your appearance will preclude you from resuming your normal activities almost immediately. Bruising may last a week, and swelling may last a month.

Fat injections, including harvesting of your fat, cost an average of $1,000 per session ($1,600 per session in New York). Multiple sessions may be required.

In summary, fat injections can be effective and lasting when injected into fat, when performed by experienced surgeons, and when over-injected to compensate for future shrinkage. But, when injected for wrinkles, the results have been disappointing.

Botox

Dynamic wrinkles, such as crow's feet, frown lines, and forehead wrinkles, are due to repetitive facial expression. Weakening the responsible muscles can improve or eliminate these wrinkles. This can be accomplished without detracting from your facial expressiveness. In 1997, plastic surgeons began using Botox injections to improve or eliminate facial wrinkles. Botox, derived from bacteria that cause botulism, has been used for decades in the medical arena. It can restore normal voice for people with a vocal chord condition called spasmodic dysphonia. It has also been used to treat uncontrollable eye twitches and to treat embarrassing sweating of the palms and underarms.

Botox can be injected by your plastic surgeon in the office. You may experience brief, mild discomfort as you are being injected. Following injection, recovery is immediate. A few experience mild bruising, which improves within a few days. You will begin to see improvement in your wrinkles within 24 hours and continue to see improvement for one week. Most

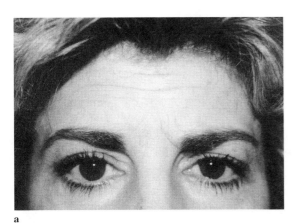
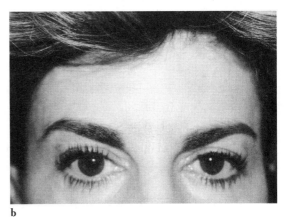

a   b

(a) Before Botox injection of forehead wrinkles and frown lines (between the eyebrows). (b) After Botox injection of forehead wrinkles and frown lines (between the eyebrows).

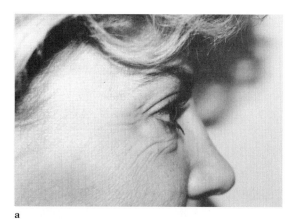 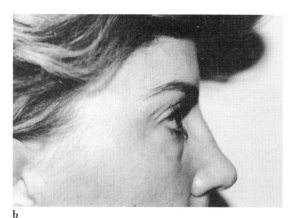

a   b

(a) Before Botox injection of crow's feet. (b) After Botox injection of crow's feet.

plastic surgeons will ask you to return in one week for a touch-up injection to ensure that your response is adequate and symmetric.

Areas most amenable to Botox are the forehead, frown lines between the eyebrows, crow's feet, lips, and neck. Results may last 2 to 12 months, and the average duration of effect is 4 to 6 months.

Cost

Your surgeon's cost of a vial of Botox is $400. One vial contains more than enough Botox to meet your needs. Your surgeon may charge you as little as $500 per session, or as much as $2,000 per session. (If you receive your injection in New York, expect to pay 50 percent more.) Expect to pay this amount every four to six months to maintain your result.

Risks

No negative long-term effects have been observed. Very few short-term problems have arisen. Risk of allergic reaction is extremely small. If Botox is injected too close to your upper eyelids, temporary upper eyelid droop may result. This can take months to improve. Injection of your forehead will diminish your ability to raise your eyebrows. This is not a problem for most, but those with marked eyebrow droop may find that their droop worsens following injection.

HELEN, *a 65-year-old department store manager, had deep forehead wrinkles, flat low eyebrows, and scowl lines. She wanted to try Botox. One week later, she returned with greatly improved forehead lines and exceedingly low eyebrows. After the Botox wore off, she had a forehead lift with good results. She still has Botox injections, but because of her lift, she no longer has low brow position.*

Satisfaction

Satisfaction following Botox injections is high, as long as the recipients understand that benefits are temporary.

Concluding Thoughts

Because of skin care's simplicity, safety, low cost, and advantage of home application, every woman should participate in a physician-supervised skin care program. The improvement in skin appearance is reliable, and the cost is affordable

Meanwhile, physician supervised micro peels and superficial peels have become immensely popular because of their simplicity, safety, effectiveness, and low cost. Here too, the benefits are great, the risks negligible, and the cost affordable.

Of the multiple options for filling wrinkles, none have proved to be lasting. If you choose to have your wrinkles filled, you should anticipate the need for ongoing treatments.

If you have had collagen injection and have been disappointed by the transient results, you may wish to try again using one of the newer alternatives to bovine collagen. These substances appear to last longer than bovine collagen, but because they have only been used since the mid-1990s, their long-term results will not be known for decades.

Finally, Botox injection is a powerful treatment because of its dramatic effect and immediate recovery. It is rapidly becoming one of the most requested procedures in plastic surgery.

In short, if you have problems with skin texture, complexion, vitality, discoloration, and wrinkles, you need not commit yourself to an expensive procedure or lengthy recovery. Each of the simple solutions offers advantages, but their effects are less potent and shorter lived than those of the serious solutions discussed in the next chapter.

Questions to Ask Your Plastic Surgeon

What treatment do you recommend and why?

Will the treatment you recommend need to be repeated?

How long do the proposed injections usually last?

How many injections do you think I will need to accomplish my goal?

How long will it take to achieve my peak result and how long will it last?

Does the fee for Botox injection include the cost of the Botox and a touch-up injection one week later?

Tips and Traps

Enroll in a skin care program through your plastic surgeon's office. It is simple, safe, effective, and economical.

Skin care specialists and plastic surgeons find most department store skin care products to be little effective. Do not be misled by promises of effectiveness if the product is not recommended by your physician.

Avoid unprotected sun exposure for at least three to six months following skin treatments. Sun protection factor (SPF) 15–30 is usually adequate.

Beware laypeople who offer chemical peels.

Decide what bothers you most about your skin, and seek a treatment that addresses your primary concern.

12

Smoothing Your Wrinkles with Serious Solutions

Medium and Deep Chemical Peels, Dermabrasion, and Laser Resurfacing

*T*o select an appropriate treatment for your skin, you and your surgeon must identify your problems, determine your goals, and define an acceptable recovery period. To help define your problems, read the section "Identify Your Skin Problems" in Chapter 11.

If you have aged and sun-damaged skin, you may seek greater improvement than is available through the simple solutions described in Chapter 11. The serious solutions described in this chapter will provide you with more dramatic and durable results. As you might expect, they also cost more, impose a period of recovery, and confer greater risks.

Chemical peels, laser, and dermabrasion are all guided by the same principles. Each treatment causes controlled injury to your skin's damaged superficial cells. Your skin then sheds those cells, allowing the healthier deep cells to surface while they are still young and fresh. Each of these treatments organizes and accelerates the process of skin turnover and helps you reclaim the skin of your youth. (Skin care and micro peels are also guided by these principles, although their effects are less profound.)

Despite the similarities of chemical peels, laser, and dermabrasion, each treatment option works to a different depth and therefore yields a different degree of improvement. No one treatment solves all problems. In general, deeper treatments yield greater

GLENDA, *a 44-year-old socialite, has battled skin problems for as long as she can remember. During her 20s, she underwent multiple dermabrasion sessions—the only option at that time—for treatment of her acne scars. During her 30s, she had several medium chemical peels to brighten her complexion, smooth her skin, and soften some of her fine wrinkles. During her 40s, she has pursued laser resurfacing for her increasingly problematic complexion and deeper wrinkles.*

improvement but impose longer recovery. Many women employ two treatment options that complement one another, such as laser resurfacing and Botox injections. (See Table 11-1, titled "Treatment Options" in Chapter 11.)

All of the treatments in this chapter, with the exception of deep peels, may need to be performed more than once to achieve optimal results. Dermabrasion, medium chemical peels, and laser may require a total of one to four treatments at six-month intervals to achieve your desired result.

Complications

When your procedure is performed by a qualified plastic surgeon, your recovery will likely be uneventful. Even in ideal circumstances, however, compli-

Safe Treatment Depth

Many women ask if their desired results can be achieved through one deep treatment rather than multiple shallower ones. Unfortunately, when dealing with dermabrasion, medium peels, and laser treatments, a single very deep treatment may result in scarring, discoloration, or both.

Each treatment may be performed to a certain safe depth (fig. 12-1). If treatment to this depth results in resolution of wrinkles and acne scars, then you need no more treatments. If your wrinkles are deeper, then you may need multiple treatments to achieve your desired result. If treatment is carried deeper than the level of safety, then scarring or discoloration may result. Deep peels illustrate this point. Although the deep peel results in overwhelming improvement in wrinkles, it permanently causes the treated skin to look bleached.

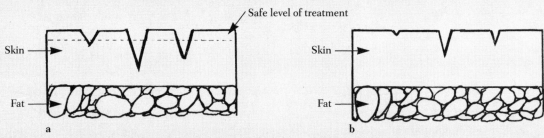

FIGURE 12-1: *Cross section of skin. (a) Before treatment, showing wrinkles and acne scars are lower than the surrounding skin. The dotted line shows the safe level of treatment. (If treatment is carried deeper, permanent scarring may result.) (b) After treatment, wrinkles and scars are shallower following treatment with dermabrasion, deep chemical peel, or laser. Because all of these wrinkles are deeper than the line of safety, one treatment will not eradicate them without causing scars. Therefore, multiple treatments are necessary. After each treatment, the deep layer of skin thickens, and the wrinkles become shallower.*

cations may occur. Chemical peels, dermabrasion, and laser treatments all may discolor skin, increase sensitivity to the sun, scar the skin, or trigger an outbreak of cold sores.

Dark Discoloration

Dark discoloration, or *hyperpigmentation*, appears as dark, blotchy, irregular patches of skin in the treated area. It may develop within several weeks of your treatment and may last for weeks or months. It is usually not permanent. Hyperpigmentation may be both prevented and treated by topical bleaching agents (see "skin care" in Chapter 11).

Women with olive or dark skin are at highest risk for dark discoloration. Many of these skin treatments are not recommended for those with dark skin. Birth control pills, antidepressants, and tetracycline may all predispose your skin to dark discoloration.

Increased Sun Sensitivity

Following chemical peel, laser, or dermabrasion, you must protect your skin from the harmful effects of the sun for at least six months. These skin treatments sensitize your skin so that minimal sun exposure may cause severe burn or dark discoloration. The already high risk is even higher if sunlight strikes unprotected skin that is still red from treatment.

Sunscreen with sun protection factor (SPF) 15 or higher is recommended. Its importance cannot be overstated. If you are unwilling or unable to avoid the sun or wear sunblock, you should not have these treatments.

Light Discoloration

Light discoloration, or *hypopigmentation*, appears as blotchy, irregular patches of skin that are lighter than the surrounding skin. It may develop within several weeks of your treatment and may last only temporarily. Risk of developing hypopigmentation is highest in those with light skin and in those receiving deep treatments.

Scarring

The deeper the treatment, the greater is its effectiveness. Yet, if performed too deeply, any procedure may cause permanent scarring. Your surgeon will try to balance giving you the greatest effect with the least risk of scarring.

If you have had radiation treatments to your face, you will be at higher risk for scarring. Your surgeon can perform a spot test with the laser or chemical peel to determine your skin's response in a tiny area. If healing is poor, it may leave a small scar. If healing is uncomplicated, you may then have your entire face treated.

If you take Accutane, an oral acne medication, you must defer chemical peels, laser resurfacing, and dermabrasion for at least one year. Accutane slows healing and predisposes to scarring.

Cold Sore Outbreak

These skin treatments may trigger a cold sore outbreak with resultant scarring especially if you have ever had cold sores. Taking antiviral medication prior to and following your treatment will reduce your risk. Defer your skin treatment until any active sores have healed.

Milia

Milia are skin eruptions that appear as tiny whiteheads. When they occur, they may do so throughout the treated area and appear quite obvious and unattractive. Because they are raised, they are not easily concealed with makeup. They may last weeks or months. Fortunately, this undesirable problem is uncommon.

Medium Chemical Peels

Medium chemical peels are highly effective in promoting skin smoothness and vitality. They also improve superficial discoloration (such as age spots) and eliminate fine wrinkles. They improve color, freshness, texture, and skin tone. They may improve blotches and can sometimes improve dark circles under your eyes. They do nothing for acne scarring or dynamic wrinkles.

To achieve the best results, two or more peels may be needed, three months apart.

Unlike deep peels, medium peels may be performed safely on people with olive and light brown skin. They may also be used in some people with dark brown skin, although the risk of discoloration is higher.

Medium depth peels can be achieved with a variety of chemicals. TCA (trichloroacetic acid) is the most common. Jessner's solution, glycolic acid, salicylic acid, and other agents are also used.

The type of chemical alone does not determine the depth of a peel. Its strength and the technique of application also matter. For example, glycolic acid used in

SUE, *a 49-year-old manicurist, had been using skin care products and micro peels for three years. While pleased with her results, she wanted a more dramatic effect. She had a five-day weekend approaching in which she could recover from a medium peel. A TCA peel provided her with the improvement she sought and allowed her to return to work with makeup in six days.*

low concentration may produce a micro peel, but used in high concentration may yield a medium peel.

Preparation

Preparing your skin prior to a medium chemical peel will result in deeper penetration, faster recovery, lower risk of discoloration, and a better result. Apply retin-A, glycolic acid, and bleaching agents daily for four to six weeks. Retin-A will help your dead superficial layers of skin shed and so will allow a chemical peel agent to penetrate more deeply. Retin-A will also stimulate your skin to regenerate and heal more quickly. Alpha hydroxy acids, such as glycolic acid, will enhance the effects of retin-A. Women with dark skin are at increased risk for developing blotchy skin after a medium chemical peel; bleaching agents used before (and after) your peel will minimize this problem. If you are on a skin care program, you may already be prepared for a medium chemical peel.

Some physicians may perform medium peels in patients who do not prepare their skin. If so, the results may not be as dramatic, recovery may be longer, and risk of discoloration is greater.

What to Expect

The Procedure

Medium peels are performed as office procedures and require 15–60 minutes. Your surgeon may offer you pain pills or sedatives to help you tolerate intense burning during peeling agent application. Your surgeon will apply a chemical solution, usually TCA, to your skin, one area at a time. When the desired depth has been achieved, your physician will neutralize the peel by applying iced saline. After ice is applied, you will have no further discomfort. Burning lasts about 2 to 10 minutes. Once all areas have been neutralized, your skin will return to its normal color in 15 to 45 minutes. To keep your skin moist and promote healing, your face will be covered with an oil-based ointment, steroid ointment, or vegetable shortening. You will then be allowed to go home.

Recovery

There will be no discomfort following the procedure. Wash your face twice daily with gentle soap and water followed by application of ointment. Your face will initially appear red. Within a few days, your superficial layers of skin will turn dark, become stiff, and resemble leather. They will then crack, flake, and peel. Flaking is usually complete in four to seven days. There will be no open wounds and no scabs.

Once your old skin has sloughed, your new skin will be bright and flushed. After your skin has finished peeling, you may begin wearing makeup. You will physically be able to resume normal activity immediately, but your appearance may preclude this. Most are able to comfortably return to public within seven days. You should resume skin care within two weeks of your procedure. Your flushed appearance will fade slowly over several weeks.

Cost

Total cost of a full-face medium chemical peel averages $2,000. If you wish to have only a portion of your face peeled, such as the area around your mouth or the area around your eyes, you will pay about $1,200. (Expect to pay 50 percent more in New York.)

Duration of Results

Medium chemical peels will last six months to two years. If you use skin care products regularly after your peel, you will extend the duration of improvement. Most women who choose medium chemical peels as the mainstay of their facial rejuvenation have a repeat peel every 6 to 12 months.

Satisfaction

Women who seek dramatically increased skin vitality with a reduction of fine wrinkles are generally satisfied with medium chemical peels, as long as they understand recovery and duration of the results, and if they do not expect improvement in dynamic wrinkles.

Deep Chemical Peels

When people speak of deep chemical peels, they are usually referring to *phenol peels*. Phenol is a caustic chemical compound. Because phenol pene-

LOUISE, *a 69-year-old with marked wrinkles around her mouth and very light skin, wanted to improve her wrinkles in a single treatment. Because she had light skin, she was a good candidate for deep peel. The peel was performed around her mouth only. She had dramatic improvement in her wrinkles, and she looked natural because of her inherently pale complexion.*

trates deeply into skin, its effects are overwhelming. Wrinkles are markedly improved and in many cases eliminated. Lax skin is tightened. Unfortunately, phenol peels pose some striking disadvantages.

Advantages

Deep chemical peel is considered the gold standard for wrinkle improvement. Results are unquestionably superior to those following other peels, laser, or dermabrasion. Just one treatment is required and results are lasting. You will continue to look younger decades after your deep chemical peel. No special preparation is necessary, and no special care is required to maintain your results afterward. Phenol peels will improve superficial acne scars and nearly all dark discoloration.

Deep peels may provide protection from skin cancer. Physicians who perform many phenol peels have noted that their patients, despite significant previous sun exposure, do not develop skin cancers. This benefit has not been proved, but the possibility is intriguing. Further research is needed. (For the present, you should not have a deep chemical peel in order to prevent or treat skin cancer.)

Disadvantages

The main disadvantage of phenol is permanent skin pallor. After your redness has faded, your face will gradually turn ghostly white, which is irreversible, unnatural, and serves as a telltale sign. You may attempt to camouflage your

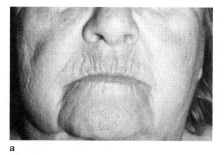 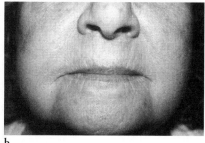

a   b

(a) Before deep chemical peel of the skin around the mouth. (b) After deep chemical peel of the skin around the mouth.

appearance with makeup, but even heavy foundation will be inadequate.

There is no way to smoothly transition from peeled to nonpeeled skin, so a clear line of demarcation will exist. The peeled area will appear white and the non-peeled skin will be your natural skin color. The point at which your peel is stopped must be chosen carefully. If your full face is peeled, the peel will be stopped about an inch below the border of your jaw. If only the area around your mouth is peeled, the peel will be performed up to your nose, down to your chin, and out to your cheek creases on either side of your mouth. The cheek creases will help conceal the line of demarcation. (If you want a deep chemical peel of your crow's feet only, you should reconsider because there are no natural skin creases in which to hide the color transition. This would result in the areas around your eyes appearing as patches of white with darker surrounding skin.)

Because of the significant alteration in skin color, deep phenol peels are suited best to those with fair skin. They are not appropriate for women with olive, brown, or black skin, as they will cause permanent disfigurement.

Your skin will never tan after a deep chemical peel. If you choose to tan the remainder of your body, an even greater discrepancy will exist between your previously peeled and non-peeled skin.

LEXY, a 63-year-old grandmother with a pale complexion, wears turtlenecks year-round. She had had a phenol chemical peel years ago, resulting in removal of all of her freckles. Because the peel stopped at her jawline, the freckles of her neck and chest remained. She was extremely self-conscious of her freckled neck compared to her freckle-free face. This sharp contrast was eye-catching and clearly unnatural. Unfortunately, the results of her deep peel were permanent. Her facial freckles could not be restored. Performing a deep peel on her neck would be medically ill-advised because the neck does not heal consistently following a phenol peel. It would also offer little improvement because it would only move the line of demarcation further down. Her freckle-free neck would then sharply contrast with her freckled chest and back. Unfortunately, nothing will solve her problem.

Phenol peels cannot be safely performed on the neck, chest, or extremities. Skin in these areas is not equipped to heal following a deep peel and is prone to scarring. Spot application is usually safe but leaves obvious white spots.

Deep chemical peels remove freckles permanently. If you are heavily freckled and have a full-face deep peel, your neck and chest will continue to be heavily freckled. Your face will be freckle-free, creating unnatural disharmony. Deep peels are not recommended for those who are heavily freckled.

Phenol must be applied slowly to one section of the face at a time. If it is applied too quickly, it can cause dangerous heart rhythms. Your heart rhythm should always be monitored during phenol application.

Because deep chemical peels may cause significant contraction of your skin, they can pull down your lower eyelids, especially if your lids are lax prior to your peel. Dry eye syndrome may result (see Chapter 4). Tightening your lower eyelid through a canthopexy procedure before your phenol peel can prevent this complication.

What to Expect

Phenol peels are performed under sedation or general anesthesia. You will be allowed to go home the same day, but will not be able to drive yourself. Discomfort is variable and will be controlled with prescription pain medication. Your skin will heal within 10 days, and you will be presentable in public with makeup in two weeks. Your final result will be evident after redness fades, approximately two or three months.

Vital Statistics

PHENOL PEEL

Anesthesia: General or heavy sedation.

Location of operation: Office or hospital.

Length of surgery: 15–60 minutes.

Length of stay: Outpatient (home same day).

Discomfort: Mild to severe. Anticipate 0–5 days of prescription pain medication.

Swelling: Moderate to severe and may temporarily interfere with eye opening. It will improve over 7–10 days.

Dressings: Two methods of dressing are used: open or closed. If open method is used, your treated skin will be covered with ointment and you will be instructed to wash your face and apply ointment beginning the day following your peel. If closed method is used, your peeled areas will be covered with tape or a flexible adherent mask immediately following the peel. You will return to your plastic surgeon's office within a few days to have the mask removed. You will then begin to wash and apply ointment twice daily. Most patients prefer the closed method because it is less messy and less painful.

The peeling process: Your face will be swollen, red, oozing, and crusted. Your face will become stiff and dark, then your skin cells will dry and begin to flake. You will be advised to not pick at your flaking skin, and you will be advised to limit your facial expressions to avoid premature peeling. Within 7 to 10 days peeling and flaking will be complete, and you will be left with healthy, smooth, bright red skin. This sunburned appearance will take two or three months to improve. Thereafter, your skin will appear extremely pale.

Makeup: May be worn about 4 days after your skin has finished peeling and flaking. Expect 10–14 days after the procedure.

Presentable in public: You will be presentable in 10–14 days with makeup.

Work: You may feel capable of returning within 3 days, but your appearance will be the limiting factor.

Exercise: May be resumed as soon as your skin has finished peeling. Expect 7–10 days.

Sun protection: SPF 15 or higher should be worn indefinitely.

Final result: Seen after your redness fades. Expect 2–3 months.

To help you plan for and recover from your procedure, reread Steps 7 and 10 of Chapter 1.

Telltale Signs

All recipients of phenol chemical peels will have a ghostly white complexion in the treated area. This permanent change in skin color is the hallmark of phenol chemical peels.

Cost

The fee for a full-face phenol peel is about $4,000. A phenol peel around the mouth only costs about $2,000. (If you plan to have your peel in New York, expect to pay about 50 percent more.) The above costs include anesthesia, operating room, and surgeon's fees.

Duration of Results

One phenol chemical peel will be lasting. Although you may redevelop fine wrinkles over time, they will not be as deep or as numerous as your original wrinkles.

Satisfaction

Women with pale skin who have profound sun damage gain dramatic improvement with phenol peels and are commonly pleased with their results. Because their change in appearance is overwhelming and because bleaching of their skin is not obvious against their pale complexion, these women are satisfied. Women with less sun damage and those with medium or dark complexions are likely to be highly dissatisfied with the results of a phenol peel, due to permanent pallor.

Dermabrasion

Dermabrasion involves using a motor-driven burr to remove superficial skin through a process that is similar to sanding. The removal of superficial skin allows healthier skin cells to surface and results in smoother texture and tighter skin.

Surgeons use their experience to determine depth of treatment; this is critical to achieving good results. If your surgeon abrades your skin too deeply, you may scar. If your treatment is too superficial, your improvement may be only slight.

Acne Scars

Acne scars, like wrinkles, are visible mostly because they are lower or deeper than surrounding skin. Light casts shadows into acne scars. If acne scars can be brought to the same level as surrounding skin, their visibility will diminish because shadows will be less obvious. This can be accomplished by either raising each scar or lowering the surrounding skin. Because raising each scar is not feasible, lowering the surrounding skin is the goal. This can be accomplished through dermabrasion or laser resurfacing.

Effectiveness of Dermabrasion

Dermabrasion is somewhat effective in improving wrinkles and acne scars, but it is not a miracle cure. Each treatment can improve acne scarring by 25 to 50 percent. Therefore, up to four treatments may be required to achieve your desired result (fig. 12-1). The greatest effect is usually achieved with the first treatment. Once acne scars are treated, the improvement is permanent, unless further acne eruptions evolve. Some acne scars may remain, even following multiple treatments.

Advantages

Some surgeons consider dermabrasion to be the treatment of choice for upper lip wrinkles and acne scars. No skin preparation is necessary prior to dermabrasion. Dermabrasion moderately improves wrinkles, acne scars, and discoloration. Postoperative swelling is milder than that following carbon dioxide laser treatment.

Disadvantages

Although dermabrasion can improve wrinkles, it is not nearly as effective as a deep chemical peel. Several dermabrasion treatments may be required. There are risks of scarring and color change, as with medium chemical peel and laser treatments, but the risk of hypopigmentation is higher. Some surgeons consider carbon dioxide or erbium laser to be better than dermabrasion for wrinkles and acne scars.

What to Expect

Dermabrasion is commonly performed under sedation anesthesia. You will be allowed to go home the same day. Discomfort is moderate and will be controlled with prescription pain medication. Your skin will heal in 7 to 10 days, and you will be presentable in public with the help of makeup within two weeks. Your redness will fade in four to six weeks, when your final result will be evident.

To help you to plan for and recover from your procedure, reread Steps 7 and 10 of Chapter 1.

Telltale Signs

Dermabrasion usually leaves no telltale signs, except in some cases when the treated area develops light discoloration, as described earlier in this chapter.

Cost

The United States average cost for full-face dermabrasion is $4,000. If you have acne scars and want only your cheeks treated, expect to pay about $3,000. If you want only your lips treated, expect to pay about $1,500. (If you plan to have dermabrasion in New York, plan to pay 50 percent more.) The above costs include anesthesia, operating room, and surgeon's fees.

Duration of Results

Dermabrasion can have a lasting effect on acne scars. Fine wrinkle improvement can be maintained through

---

Vital Statistics

DERMABRASION

Anesthesia: General or sedation.

Location of operation: Office or hospital.

Length of surgery: 15–60 minutes.

Length of stay: Outpatient (home same day).

Discomfort: Moderate. Anticipate 3–7 days of prescription pain medication.

Swelling: Will last for 7–14 days.

Dressings: Ointment and bandages will be applied. You will be instructed to wash your face daily and reapply ointment until your skin has healed. Expect 7–10 days. After your skin heals, it will appear sunburned. It will return to its natural color in 4–6 weeks.

Makeup: May be worn shortly after your skin heals.

Presentable in public: You will be presentable with makeup in 7–10 days.

Work: You may feel capable of returning within 3 days, but your appearance will be the limiting factor.

Exercise: May be resumed within a week.

Sun protection: SPF 15 or higher for 3–6 months.

Final result: Seen in 4–6 weeks.

TAMMY, *a 45-year-old woman whose twin daughters recently left for college, wanted to reward herself for surviving their adolescence. She had researched the carbon dioxide laser and thought it would be appropriate. She wanted as dramatic a result as possible, but did not want the pallor caused by phenol peels. Recovery time was not a concern. Following just one carbon dioxide laser treatment, her wrinkles were improved to her satisfaction.*

skin care. Dynamic wrinkles, because they are caused by ongoing muscle activity, will redevelop within one to five years.

Satisfaction

Satisfaction following dermabrasion varies depending on the severity of the problem. The deeper the wrinkles and acne scars, the less likely dermabrasion will yield a satisfactory result, and the more likely that multiple treatments will be required. Those who expect more from dermabrasion than it can deliver will be disappointed.

Carbon Dioxide Laser Resurfacing

A laser is a powerful beam of light that can vaporize the top layers of skin. Deeper, healthier cells then replace the superficial cells that were vaporized. Lasers also promote reorganization of collagen, which is the "meat" of the skin. Its reorganization results in diminished wrinkles and improved skin tone. Fine wrinkles will be removed altogether. Other benefits include

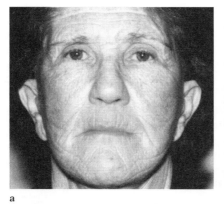
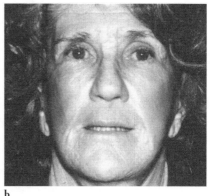

a   b

(a) Before carbon dioxide laser treatment of full face. (b) After carbon dioxide laser treatment of full face.

Printed with permission from Robert M. Adrian, M.D., F.A.C.S., Center for Laser Surgery, Washington, D.C.

improved skin texture, smoothness, and freshness. Superficial discoloration can also be improved.

Dynamic wrinkles—those associated with smiling, laughing, and frowning—will eventually recur because facial expression will continue. You can expect about 50 to 80 percent improvement in laugh line wrinkles with each treatment. Depending on the severity of your wrinkles, one to three treatments may be necessary. They may be performed as soon as six months apart. Those with deeper wrinkles may require up to four treatments. You will see the most dramatic improvement after your first treatment.

Advantages

Carbon dioxide laser resurfacing moderately improves wrinkles without the bleaching changes typical of deep chemical peels. It also improves discoloration and acne scars. If the skin has been adequately prepared with bleaching agents, carbon dioxide laser resurfacing can be performed safely on those with olive skin. It should not be used on brown or black skin because of the high risk of permanent skin color changes.

Laser resurfacing promotes skin contraction, which improves skin tone. Although laser resurfacing is not a substitute for facelift, some women are able to defer facelifts for a few more years after laser resurfacing.

Disadvantages

The greatest disadvantage of carbon dioxide laser resurfacing is the lengthy recovery. The skin may take 10 days or longer to heal. Swelling may persist for weeks, and redness may persist for months. For these reasons, carbon dioxide laser resurfacing is sought mainly by those who can afford to take two weeks away from work and social events.

Laser resurfacing does not approach the overwhelming and lasting improvement in wrinkles that is possible with one deep chemical peel. Laser resurfacing causes blotchy discoloration in 5 to 10 percent of patients. Most

---

Synonyms for Carbon Dioxide Laser Resurfacing

Plastic surgeons use many terms to describe laser resurfacing of the face. Some of these terms are unfortunately also used to describe erbium laser resurfacing, which, as you will see, is quite different.

Laser CO_2	*Laser desurfacing*
CO_2 laser	*Lasabrasion*
Laser vaporization	*Wrinkle laser*
Laser resurfacing	*Laser peeling*

The carbon dioxide laser was so named because, in it, carbon dioxide is used to convert light into a laser beam. (Other substances, such as helium, argon, krypton, xenon, and erbium are used in the lasers for which they are named.)

discoloration fades within six weeks, but it may last up to a year. The darker your skin, the greater your chance of discoloration. Carbon dioxide laser is therefore not well suited to those with brown or black skin. And the more sun exposure you receive afterward, the greater your risk of discoloration. Preparation of your skin with bleaching agents can minimize skin discoloration.

Because laser resurfacing tightens your skin, it may pull down your lower eyelids if they have poor skin tone (see Chapter 4). Contraction of the lower eyelids may occur in 1 to 5 percent of those treated. This may or may not require surgery, called *canthopexy*, for correction. Your surgeon should approach laser resurfacing of your lower eyelid cautiously.

Facial spider veins may develop in 2 or 3 percent of patients. These veins may later be treated with another laser.

Preparation

Retin-A, glycolic acid, and bleaching agents—available through your skin care specialist or plastic surgeon—will help prepare your skin for laser resurfacing. They will reduce your risk of discoloration, speed healing, and boost your cosmetic result. Use these products consistently for at least six weeks prior to your procedure.

The Procedure

After you are sedated, your eyes and teeth will be covered with protective guards. Your surgeon will then apply the laser beam over an entire section of your face, wipe away the vaporized superficial skin layer, and repeat this process to the appropriate depth.

What to Expect

Carbon dioxide laser resurfacing is most commonly performed under heavy sedation or general anesthesia. You will be allowed to go home the same day. Discomfort is mild to severe. Your skin will heal in 7–10 days, and you will be presentable in public with makeup in two weeks. Your final result will be evident within three months.

To help you plan for and recover from your procedure, reread Steps 7 and 10 of Chapter 1.

Vital Statistics

CARBON DIOXIDE LASER RESURFACING

Anesthesia: *General or sedation.*

Location of operation: *Office or hospital.*

Length of surgery: *15–60 minutes.*

Length of stay: *Outpatient (home same day).*

Discomfort: *Variable depending on the dressing placed at the time of your procedure. Anticipate 2–7 days of prescription pain medication.*

Swelling: *Moderate to severe and lasts 1–3 weeks.*

Dressings: *Treated areas will appear as abrasions. They will weep, ooze, and hurt when uncovered. To facilitate healing and minimize discomfort, your treated skin may be covered with a masklike dressing that will spontaneously lift off within a few days. Alternatively, ointment may be applied. Most patients prefer the mask dressing, which is neater and involves less discomfort.*

Healing: *Your skin will heal in 7–10 days and will then appear sunburned. Redness will improve over 1–3 months, depending on the depth of your treatment. Those who have had deep laser resurfacing for significant wrinkle improvement will have persistent redness. Those who have more superficial resurfacing will have faster resolution of their redness.*

Makeup: *May be worn in 2 weeks.*

Presentable in public: *You will be presentable with makeup in 10–14 days.*

Work: *You may feel capable of returning within 3–5 days, but your appearance will be the limiting factor.*

Exercise: *May be resumed in 2 weeks.*

Sun protection: *SPF 15 or higher for 3–6 months.*

Resume skin care: *You may resume skin care products after your skin has healed.*

Final result: *Will be seen after your redness has faded, approximately 1–3 months.*

Telltale Signs

Carbon dioxide laser usually leaves no telltale signs, unless the treated area develops discoloration, as described earlier in this chapter.

Cost

The United States average cost for full face carbon dioxide laser resurfacing is $4,200. The total cost for treating one part of your face, such as the areas around your eyes, the areas around your mouth, or your cheeks averages $2,000. (If you plan to have this procedure in New York, expect to pay 50 percent more.) The above costs include anesthesia, operating room, and surgeon's fees.

Duration of Results

Carbon dioxide laser will have lasting effects on acne scars. Wrinkles, because they are caused by ongoing muscle activity, will redevelop within one to five years.

Satisfaction

Women who have carbon dioxide laser resurfacing are typically satisfied with their results, provided that they understand the lengthy recovery period. Those who expect brief recovery or who have unrealistic expectations will be dissatisfied.

Erbium Laser

The erbium laser was developed in response to demands for effective skin treatments with rapid recovery. The erbium laser and carbon dioxide laser share some similarities, but the greatest difference is that the erbium laser does not heat skin while vaporizing it. There is less thermal damage to the remaining skin and thus faster recovery. The skin heals in 4 to 7 days, and redness lasts for 10 days to 2 weeks.

Regarding the effectiveness of the erbium laser, plastic surgeons debate. Most surgeons think the erbium laser yields a 40–60 percent improvement in dynamic wrinkles with each treatment, which is slightly less than the carbon dioxide laser. The erbium laser may be necessary one to four times at four to six month intervals for peak results.

Unlike the carbon dioxide laser, the erbium laser has been used with reliable results in people with

COLLEEN, a 45-year-old lawyer, helped her best friend recover from carbon dioxide laser resurfacing. She wanted similar results but could not afford two weeks to recover. She chose erbium laser treatments with the understanding that her wrinkle reduction would be less impressive. Following one treatment, she had reasonable improvement in her wrinkles and was back to work in six days.

olive, brown, and black skin. It may also fade discoloration, reduce acne scars, and improve skin tone. One additional benefit is that an anesthesiologist is not usually required for erbium treatment. Thus, the total cost may be lower than that for carbon dioxide laser treatment.

What to Expect

Erbium laser is commonly performed with little or no sedation, and you will be allowed to go home the same day. Discomfort is mild. Your skin will heal in four to seven days, and you will be presentable in public with makeup in one week. Your final result will be evident in two weeks.

To help you to plan for and recover from your procedure, reread Steps 7 and 10 of Chapter 1.

Telltale Signs

Erbium laser usually leaves no telltale signs, unless the treated area develops discoloration, as described earlier in this chapter.

Cost

A full-face erbium laser treatment costs an average of $3,400 in the United States. Treatment of part of your face, such as the area around your eyes or the area around your mouth, will cost about $1,700. (Expect to pay 50 percent more in New York.)

Duration of Results

Erbium laser will have lasting effects on acne scars. Dynamic wrinkles, because they are caused by ongoing muscle activity, will redevelop within one to five years.

Synonyms for Erbium Laser Resurfacing

Plastic surgeons use many terms to describe laser resurfacing of the face. Some of these terms are unfortunately also used to describe carbon dioxide laser resurfacing, which is quite different from the erbium laser.

Erbium-YAG laser	*Laser desurfacing*
Erbium laser	*Lasabrasion*
Laser vaporization	*Wrinkle laser*
Laser resurfacing	*Laser peeling*

The erbium laser was so named because, in it, the chemical element erbium is used to convert light into a laser beam.

Vital Statistics

ERBIUM LASER RESURFACING

Anesthesia: Topical or sedation.

Location of operation: Office or hospital.

Length of surgery: 30–60 minutes.

Length of stay: Outpatient (home same day).

Discomfort: Mild. Anticipate 0–2 days of prescription pain medication.

Swelling: Improves in 3–7 days.

Dressing: Your treated areas will weep, ooze, and hurt when exposed to air. To facilitate healing and minimize discomfort, your treated skin may be covered with a masklike dressing that will spontaneously lift off within a few days. Alternatively, ointment may be applied. Most patients prefer the masklike dressing because it is less messy and more comfortable.

Healing: Your skin will heal in 4–7 days, and will then appear sunburned. Redness will improve over 1 to 2 weeks, depending on the depth of your treatment.

Makeup: May be worn after your skin heals.

Presentable in public: You will be presentable once you can wear makeup.

Work: You may feel capable of returning within a day, but your appearance will be the limiting factor.

Exercise: May be resumed in 1 week.

Sun protection: SPF 15 or higher for 3–6 months.

Resume skin care: You may resume skin care products after your skin has healed.

Final result: Seen in 2 weeks.

Satisfaction

Women have been satisfied with erbium laser treatment because it has offered moderately impressive results with a relatively short recovery time.

Concluding Thoughts

The solutions to the problem of aged and sun-damaged skin presented in this chapter are for women who seek dramatic change. For that, they must be willing to pay higher fees, endure longer recovery periods, and accept certain risks. The potential benefits are great, but the trade-offs must be balanced.

When compared to all simple and serious treatment options, *medium chemical peels* provide an intermediate level of improvement at an intermediate cost and impose an intermediate period of recovery. They are ideal for the woman who wants more than a superficial peel but cannot afford the expense or recovery time of a deeper treatment.

Phenol peels have the most profound effect on wrinkles and are used successfully in properly chosen patients. Because of lengthy recovery and permanent pallor, it is one of the least commonly employed treatments for wrinkled and sun-damaged skin.

Dermabrasion has been used for decades to smooth skin and reduce wrinkles and acne scars. Like most treatments for skin problems, you may need multiple sessions to achieve your desired results.

Since the advent of laser technology, many plastic surgeons have turned to lasers to achieve the same goals they once attained through dermabrasion. Other plastic surgeons maintain that dermabrasion works better. Those who tout dermabrasion are probably more experienced

Questions to Ask Your Plastic Surgeon

What treatment do you recommend and why?

How many treatments will I need?

What recovery should I anticipate?

Am I at risk for skin color changes following treatment?

Will the treatment you recommend need to be repeated?

How long will my results last?

How can I best prepare my skin for the treatment you recommend?

Tips and Traps

Avoid unprotected sun exposure for at least three to six months following any skin treatment. Sun protection factor (SPF) 15–30 is usually adequate.

Understand that plastic surgeons have not reached a clear consensus regarding the relative effectiveness of carbon dioxide laser, erbium laser, and dermabrasion. Surgeons recommend the treatment which yields the best result in their own hands, so you are encouraged to follow that recommendation.

Ask to be treated with antiviral medication prior to a medium or deep peel, dermabrasion, or laser resurfacing. This will reduce your risk of cold sore outbreak and scarring after treatment.

If you seek a phenol peel, expect your skin to become permanently pale in the area treated.

Anticipate some improvement with each treatment, but do not expect one procedure to cure all skin problems. The exception to this rule is a deep peel.

Beware potential problems with your lower eyelids following laser treatment or chemical peel.

in this technique and can achieve better results than they can with the laser. Those who promote laser are likely more experienced with it and can achieve better results than with dermabrasion. Clearly, plastic surgeons have not reached a consensus.

Carbon dioxide laser resurfacing offers moderate wrinkle improvement. However, it imposes a lengthy recovery time, which discourages many from pursuing it.

Finally *erbium laser* is capable of providing effective improvement with a relatively short recovery. Although the erbium laser is not as effective as the carbon dioxide laser in treatment of wrinkles, recovery is significantly shorter. Erbium laser is more effective than medium chemical peel, yet the recovery is about the same. For these reasons, erbium laser therapy has become one of the most popular treatments for aged and sun-damaged skin.

TABLE 12-1 *Comparison of Chemical Peels, Dermabrasion, and Laser Resurfacing*

Treatment	Micro and superficial peel	Medium chemical peel	Deep chemical peel	Derm-abrasion	Laser resurfacing with CO$_2$	Laser resurfacing with Erbium
Most common chemical used	30–50% Glycolic acid[a]	35–40% TCA[b]	Phenol	Not applicable	Not applicable	Not applicable
Effect on wrinkles	Improves fine wrinkles only	Improves fine wrinkles	Overwhelming improvement in all wrinkles	Improves fine wrinkles and dynamic wrinkles	Improves dynamic wrinkles by 50–80% after each treatment	Improves dynamic wrinkles by 40–60% after each treatment
Skin preparation prior to treatment[c]	None	4–6 weeks of retin-A, AHAs, and bleaching agents	None	None	4–6 weeks of retin-A, AHAs, and bleaching agents	4–6 weeks of retin-A, AHAs, and bleaching agents
Anesthesia	None	Oral sedative or pain pill	General anesthesia or intravenous sedation	General anesthesia or intravenous sedation	General anesthesia or intravenous sedation	Topical anesthetic, with or without sedatives
Recovery[d]	Instant	4–7 days	10–14 days	7–10 days	10–14 days	4–7 days

(continued)

Table 12-1 (*Continued*)

Treatment	Micro and superficial peel	Medium chemical peel	Deep chemical peel	Derm-abrasion	Laser resurfacing with CO_2	Laser resurfacing with Erbium
Duration of effect	Effect lessens if skin is not maintained with regular peels every 2–3 months.	Effect lessens if skin is not maintained through skin care or micro peels.	Effect is lasting. Women rarely seek more than one phenol peel.	Effect on acne scarring is permanent. Effect on wrinkles may dissipate over years.	Effect on acne scarring is permanent. Effect on wrinkles may dissipate over years.	Effect on acne scarring is permanent. Effect on wrinkles may dissipate over years.
Number of treatments needed	Every other week for three months, then every 2–3 months	One to four, at 3–6 months intervals	One	One to four, at 6 month intervals	One to four, at 6 month intervals	One to four, at 6 month intervals
Drawbacks	No impact on dynamic wrinkles; requires maintenance	No impact on dynamic wrinkles or acne scarring	Skin appears bleached permanently and will never tan. It is not for freckled individuals.	Risk of light discoloration	Lengthy recovery; redness may last for weeks or months	Not as effective as carbon dioxide laser or phenol peel
Benefits	Gradual improvement; no recovery time	Moderate improvement in complexion with relatively brief recovery time	Overwhelming impact on wrinkles after one treatment	Moderate improvement in wrinkles and acne scarring	Moderate improvement in wrinkles and acne scarring	Moderate improvement in wrinkles and acne scarring with relatively brief recovery time. Safe for women with olive or black skin
Best candidates	Women who seek general improvement in complexion but cannot afford any recovery time	Women who seek significant improvement in complexion, superficial discoloration, and fine wrinkles	Women who seek an overwhelming and lasting improvement in their wrinkles and can tolerate the permanent bleaching effect on the skin	Women who seek treatment of acne scarring and lip wrinkles	Women who seek significant improvement in wrinkles and can afford lengthy recovery	Women who seek moderate improvement dynamic wrinkles, but cannot afford lengthy recovery

(*continued*)

TABLE 12-1 *(Continued)*

TREATMENT	MICRO AND SUPERFICIAL PEEL	MEDIUM CHEMICAL PEEL	DEEP CHEMICAL PEEL	DERM-ABRASION	LASER RESURFACING WITH CO_2	LASER RESURFACING WITH ERBIUM
Cost per treatment[e]	$60–80 per micro peel and $80–120 per superficial peel	$2,000	$4,000	$4,000	$4,200	$3,400

[a]Used in 30–50 percent concentration, glycolic acid is a micro peel. Medium depth peels can be achieved with a 70% solution.

[b]TCA peel can induce a micro, medium, or deep peel, depending on its concentration, the patient's skin preparation, and the technique of application. The most common clinical use is at medium depth.

[c]The result of a medium peel will be better if the skin was prepared in advance. Recovery following medium peels and laser resurfacing will be expedited in those with properly prepared skin. Since retin-A alone is difficult for many to tolerate, it is helpful to use a combination of retin-A and a steroid cream. Preparation with a bleaching agent such as soloquin is also very helpful to prevent problems with dark discoloration in the postoperative period.

[d]Recovery time is the time required for skin to heal such that there are no open wounds and makeup can be worn. After recovery, skin may remain red for weeks or months, depending on the treatment.

[e]Cost includes surgeon's fee, operating room fee, and anesthesia fee for a full-face treatment.

13

Having Plastic Surgery During Your Lunch Hour

Treatments for Discoloration, Spider Veins, Tattoos, Unwanted Hair, Thin Lips, Stretch Marks, and Cellulite

*M*any minor problems can be improved through simple treatments. These procedures have come to be known as "lunch hour treatments," because they are relatively quick, painless, and impose little or no recovery time. Skin discolorations, such as birthmarks, freckles, melasma, age spots, and moles, can be addressed through relatively simple treatments. Spider veins of the legs and face are amenable to injections or laser therapy. Decorative tattoos can be removed, and cosmetic makeup tattoos can be placed. Growth of unwanted hair can be temporarily halted. Thin lips can be augmented. All of these things can be accomplished through office procedures that are generally safe, effective, and affordable.

Yet, these treatments are not necessarily innocuous. Many of these remedies do pose potentially serious consequences. Some treatments provide only temporary improvement, even though advertisements may state otherwise. Others may provide no improvement. Unfortunately, in the arena of minor office procedures, false claims prevail. You, as a consumer, must educate yourself so that you are not misled.

Lasers are the treatment of choice for many of these problems, so a short primer on lasers begins this chapter.

LISA, *a 42-year-old freelance artist, had a number of concerns as she prepared herself for her annual trip with her husband to Key West. She was embarrassed about spider veins around her knees and hair around her belly button. She also did not want to be bothered with daily eye-makeup application. In a short time and at a reasonable cost, she had spider veins treated, abdominal hair removed, and eyeliner tattoo placed.*

Primer on Lasers

Laser technology was developed decades ago but continues to be improved and refined. In laser therapy, a beam of light is amplified and becomes powerful when applied to particular colors or substances. (The word laser is simply an acronym for "light amplification by stimulated emission of radiation.") Various types of laser can vaporize certain kinds of tissue in a controllable manner.

Lasers are important treatment options for many minor skin problems. In the realm of plastic surgery, laser therapy is used for the treatment of wrinkles, scars, birthmarks, spider veins, skin discolorations, age spots, and tattoos.

Lasers do not vanquish all skin problems, and lasers are not appropriate for every procedure. They play a role in some cosmetic treatments, but their use must be kept in perspective. Lasers are a tool, not a panacea.

Different Lasers for Different Problems

There are as many different lasers as there are skin problems. Each laser has strengths, weaknesses, and targeted areas of effectiveness. For example, some lasers are effective for treating shades of brown and red—and are therefore used for removal of age spots, brown birthmarks, and red tattoos. Other lasers are effective for vascular problems such as spider veins, red or purple (vascular) birthmarks, and exuberant scars. Other lasers will target blue, black, and green; these may be used to remove decorative tattoos.

Two lasers, the carbon dioxide laser and the erbium laser are used to treat wrinkles and are discussed in Chapter 12. The lasers discussed in this chapter are markedly different, particularly in terms of discomfort and recovery. The lasers in this chapter are used without anesthetic, enable immediate recovery, are generally affordable, and can be performed by a nurse or technician (rather than a physician).

Laser Treatments

Laser treatments for birthmark, spider vein, tattoo, stretch mark, and hair removal are performed in the office and require no special preparation. Treatments are associated with mild discomfort, not unlike a small rubber band snapping against skin. The discomfort is well tolerated when small areas are treated, but if large areas are treated, such as in hair removal, discomfort may interfere with the procedure. Treatments usually do not require sedatives, pain medications, or injections of local anesthetic. Treatment times vary depending on the size of the area treated. A small tattoo can be treated in five minutes. Hair removal from both legs and groins may require two hours. Dressings are unnecessary, as there will be no open wounds.

Recovery

Recovery is rapid. Bruising might occur following some laser treatments and disappears in 3 to 10 days. Some lasers may cause temporary dryness, crusting, blistering, and roughness of the skin, which also improve in a few days. You will be able to resume normal activities immediately following laser treatment, but you may prefer to keep the treated areas covered with clothing until appearance is back to normal.

Skin Discoloration

Your skin may temporarily become darker or lighter than surrounding skin. If your skin is olive, brown, or black, you will be at higher risk for dark discoloration. If your skin is pale, you will be at risk for light discoloration. These dark or light areas are blotchy, irregular, and unsightly, but usually disappear within a few months. Unprotected sun exposure may trigger dark blotchy skin, so you will be advised to wear sunscreen with SPF 30 or higher for several months following laser treatment.

Scars

Permanent scarring may occur if lasers are applied too intensely or too deeply. This is rare with the lasers discussed in this chapter. One of the great advantages of laser surgery is that lasers usually leave no scars. Laser surgery may also remove all traces of the original problems while leaving no telltale signs of treatment.

Number of Treatments

The number of treatments necessary depends on your problem, its severity, your response to treatment, and your goal. Some birthmarks can be effectively treated with one or two treatments. Others require a dozen treatments. Some problems, such as unwanted hair, are only temporarily improved by laser and require routine maintenance treatments.

Cost

For birthmarks, freckles, tattoos, spider veins, hair removal, and other minor skin problems, laser treatment in the United States costs $300 to $1,500 per session with a typical fee of $700. Prices will vary depending on the type of laser used and the size of area being treated.

Skin Discolorations

Birthmarks

Birthmarks vary in color and may range from cream colored to deep purple. The most common birthmarks are called *café-au-lait* spots because of their "coffee with milk" appearance. They may increase in size and number during childhood and puberty. These birthmarks may be effectively treated with one to three laser sessions. Because they may recur following partial treatment, complete removal is recommended. Most café-au-lait spots respond well to laser treatment.

Red and purple birthmarks are composed of tiny blood vessels. These birthmarks are called *port wine stains* because their appearance is similar to spilled red wine. Port wine stains may cover much of the face. Due to their size and color, they are disfiguring and obvious. Most can be effectively treated with laser, but numerous treatments are required.

Freckles

In our culture, freckles convey innocence and immaturity. Many tire of this image as they age.

Freckles are particularly problematic in the summertime, because they increase in number and appear-

JODI, *a 25-year-old law student, was tired of her youthful appearing freckled face. She would soon be entering the professional world and thought she could little afford the look of naiveté. She underwent a medium chemical peel, her freckles faded nicely, and she was back to her usual routine within a week.*

JOSIE AND HEIDI *were friends who had both developed patches of melasma during pregnancy. The Wood's lamp revealed that Josie's melasma was superficial and Heidi's was deep. Josie's discoloration disappeared with topical bleaching agents, which she used twice daily at home (see Chapter 11). Heidi's deeper discoloration has shown little change despite multiple chemical peels.*

ance with sun exposure. Preventive measures include sun avoidance and use of sun block. Micro peels and medium peels help fade existing freckles (Chapters 11 and 12). Deep peels will permanently erase freckles. Lasers may be used for freckles, but several treatments are necessary and freckles may recur.

Melasma

Melasma is an area of dark, blotchy skin that may develop on the faces or necks of women who are pregnant or using oral contraceptives. Melasma has a distinctive appearance with irregular borders and a "dirty" appearance. This condition may be precipitated or worsened by unprotected sun exposure. Sun avoidance and strong sunscreens may prevent melasma from worsening but will probably not improve it.

Treatment of melasma depends on its depth. Your plastic surgeon can determine if your melasma is superficial or deep by shining a black light, called a *Wood's lamp*, on your skin. Superficial melasma can be remedied through superficial chemical peels, medium chemical peels, or daily application of bleaching agents (Chapters 11 and 12).

Deep melasma is more difficult to eradicate. Medium chemical peels may improve deep melasma, but the final results are neither consistent nor lasting. Even deep chemical peels may fail to correct deep melasma. Lasers offer no benefits in treatment of melasma. Unfortunately, if you have deep melasma, it may be permanent.

Age Spots

Age spots are also known as liver spots and are due to cumulative ultraviolet light exposure. As the hands, face, and chest receive the greatest sun exposure, age spots are most prevalent in these areas. Age spots, like freckles and melasma, worsen during periods of unprotected sun exposure.

Age spots can be treated with bleaching agents, chemical peels, or laser. Bleaching agents and micro peels will be effective for some superficial age spots but will not alter deeper ones. Medium peels are more effective. Deep peels are effective in treating all age spots, but they cause permanent skin bleaching, so they are not often used. Age spots are most effectively treated with two or three laser treatments. Age spots on the hands and face respond best. Age spots on the legs are difficult to improve.

Rosacea

Rosacea is a skin disorder in which the cheeks, nose, and chin become easily flushed in response to spicy foods, alcohol, or stress. After many years, the affected areas may become permanently flushed and develop small spider veins. Acne may also develop.

Rosacea occurs most commonly in middle-aged women of Celtic heritage. Laser treatments will eradicate rosacea in two or three sessions.

Moles

Moles are common skin irregularities that can be frustrating for some women. The vast majority of moles are simply small benign skin growths. Moles may be skin-colored or darker, small or large, flat or raised, hairy or bald. Most women seek to have them removed for aesthetic reasons, especially when they occur on the face. They are surprised to learn that mole removal leaves a scar.

Moles may either be shaved or excised. Shaving involves planing the mole so that it is level with the skin. It leaves a smaller scar but carries a higher risk of mole recurrence, because the mole is not removed in its entirety. Excision involves cutting the mole out in an ellipse and sewing the remaining skin together. The scar is longer, but the mole will not likely recur.

Regardless of how a mole is removed, the scar often fades and becomes undetectable. However, the final scar may be visible, and the extent of its visibility cannot be predicted. Women with moles are forced to make a decision. They may choose to keep their mole or risk a visible scar after its removal. In most cases, the scar will be less visible than the mole, and the exchange is worthwhile.

Removal of benign moles is not usually covered by insurance. The average cost is $600 for one mole. Some surgeons charge less for each subsequent mole.

LYNNE, a 46-year-old business consultant, developed rosacea in her late 30s. She tried to camouflage it with makeup but was only partially successful. Although she drank alcohol rarely, she thought rosacea gave her the appearance of an alcoholic. After three laser treatments, her rosacea was gone, as was her concern over her appearance.

MARTY, a 47-year-old woman, wanted to have a small mole removed from her chin. However, she became anxious when she found out that she would have a small scar. She said that she was consulting a plastic surgeon in order to avoid a scar. When no guarantees would be made regarding the final visibility of the scar, she chose to keep her mole.

Varicose Veins

Spider veins and varicose veins are not the same, but often occur concurrently. Varicose veins are distended veins beneath the skin. Varicose veins, like spider veins, are related to prolonged standing, female gender, pregnancy, and genetic predisposition. Each of these conditions may trigger incompetence of the valves within the veins. (Valves keep venous blood flowing in one direction— toward the heart.) If valves are incompetent, blood may back up within the vein, causing the vein to stretch, become visible, and impose aching pain. Varicose veins may appear as bluish bumps on the skin. The simplest treatments for varicose veins are support hose, leg elevation, and regular exercise. These treatments may improve minor discomfort, but will fail to alleviate significant discomfort and will not address appearance.

Those with unsightly veins and aching pain often require surgery to remove their varicose veins. Because the valves are incompetent, varicose veins are no longer functional, and their presence is not missed. (Deeper veins conduct return of blood to the heart.) As an alternative to surgery, some vascular surgeons inject varicose veins with a chemical that causes them to collapse and scar closed. General and vascular surgeons manage varicose veins; plastic surgeons usually do not.

The procedure is performed in the office with local anesthesia. You will be able to drive immediately following the procedure. Most likely your activity will not be restricted.

Your surgeon should send all moles to a pathologist for microscopic evaluation to rule out cancer. Do not try to convince your surgeon otherwise to save money. There is no way to tell if a mole is cancerous just by looking at it—it must be sent to a pathologist. The results should be available the day you return to have your stitches removed.

Spider Veins

On the Legs

One-half million spider vein treatments are performed each year in this country. Spider veins, or *telangiectasias,* are small visible vessels within the skin. They develop when deep leg veins are subjected to increased stress, such as during pregnancy or after prolonged standing (fig. 13-1). They are also more common in women with varicose veins, those who take oral contraceptive pills, and those whose mothers had spider veins.

Spider veins have no known medical consequences. Those who seek spider vein removal do so for purely cosmetic reasons.

Both Varicose and Spider Veins

If you have both spider veins and varicose veins, your varicose veins must be treated first. If your spider veins are treated first, you will be at increased risk for rapid recurrence of spider veins and matting (see "Complications"). If your varicose veins are treated first, these problems will be minimized. Also, the successful treatment of varicose veins may reduce your spider veins before they are treated.

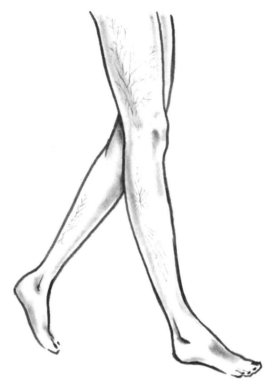

FIGURE 13-1 *Spider veins.*

Prevention

There is no proof that medical support hose prevent spider veins, although they may do so indirectly through their effects on varicose veins. (Support hose may prevent varicose veins from developing or worsening.)

Treatment

The two options for spider vein treatment are sclerotherapy and laser. They may be employed independently or in combination.

SCLEROTHERAPY

Sclerotherapy involves injecting a liquid chemical through a tiny needle directly into your spider veins, causing them to contract and collapse. The chemical may be highly concentrated salt water, a biological detergent, or a natural chemical compound. Because this technique relies upon fitting a tiny needle into a tiny vein, it is best suited to medium and large spider veins. The tiniest spider veins are difficult to treat reliably with this technique.

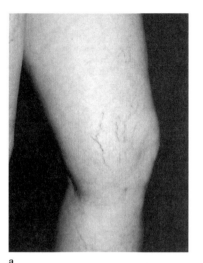
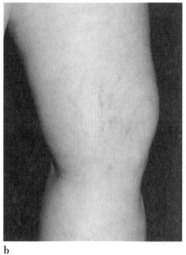
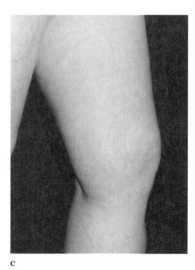

a
b
c

(a) Before sclerotherapy treatment of spider veins. (b) After first sclerotherapy treatment of spider veins. (c) After second sclerotherapy treatment of spider veins.

The procedure is performed in the office by a plastic surgeon or nurse and is relatively painless. Anesthesia is not necessary. Even those who fear needles tolerate this type of injection well, because the needles are extremely small. Because spider veins are often interconnected, like branches of a tree, a single injection at the base may cause an entire family of spider veins to collapse. Depending on the number of spider veins, the procedure may require five minutes to one hour. Afterward, you will wear ace bandages or compression hose for 3 to 10 days as recommended by your plastic surgeon. You may resume sedentary activities immediately. For best results, you should avoid exercise, hot baths, and alcohol for two or three days, because they cause blood vessel dilation, which may compromise your result.

Anticipate 50 to 90 percent improvement in spider veins following each sclerotherapy session. Some veins may fail to respond due to small vein size, lack of compression following injection, or features of the vein that you cannot control. You may need two to six sclerotherapy sessions at 6 to 12 week intervals to achieve your desired results. Understand that some small spider veins may never be successfully treated through sclerotherapy.

LASER TREATMENT

During laser treatment of spider veins, the laser is applied to the skin over your spider veins. Laser energy causes your spider veins to coagulate and shrink.

Laser therapy is most effective for small and medium size spider veins. (Large spider veins are best treated with sclerotherapy.)

Immediately following treatment, spider veins will be darker and more visible. Over two to four weeks, they will fade, although in rare cases the treated veins remain dark for six months or longer. Avoid unprotected sun for six weeks to decrease your risk of skin discoloration. Ace wraps and support hose are not necessary. You may exercise immediately. Laser treatment usually leaves no scars.

An average of three treatments will be required at three month intervals. After the first treatment, you will see a 70 to 80 percent improvement in the appearance of your spider veins, but all of them will still be visible. Each subsequent treatment results in 70 to 80 percent improvement. Compared to sclerotherapy, laser treatment offers greater improvement in small spider veins, and less improvement in large ones. Many plastic surgeons believe that, although lasers continue to improve, sclerotherapy remains the most effective way of treating spider veins.

> **RENEE**, *a 42-year-old salesperson, was in the top 100 of all salespeople in her corporation. As a result, she won a trip to Hawaii with the other top performers. She did not want her colleagues to see her spider veins. After injection of the medium and large spider veins, she underwent three laser treatments. By the time she left for the trip, there was no evidence of spider veins or of previous treatment.*

COMBINATION THERAPY

If you have small, medium, and large spider veins, you may benefit from both sclerotherapy and laser therapy. You may wish to start with sclerotherapy, because sometimes all veins will be improved after injecting the larger ones. This may reduce the number of veins that need to be treated by laser, lowering your overall cost.

Some surgeons perform sclerotherapy and laser treatment on the same day. Most treat spider veins in stages to ensure the best possible results.

Complications

When performed or supervised by a qualified plastic surgeon, your procedure and recovery will likely be uneventful. Yet, even in ideal circumstances, complications may occur.

MATTING

The sudden appearance of new spider veins, known as matting, may occur anywhere on the treated extremity. Matting occurs in 10 to 20 percent of patients following sclerotherapy and 5 to 15 percent following laser. Matting develops within one week of treatment and is most common in women who have spider veins treated in the presence of varicose veins. Obese women and those who take hormones or oral contraceptive pills are also at high risk. Matting may improve on its own but may take one year to do so. Some of the new spider veins will persist and require treatment. Persistent matting usually responds well to either laser or sclerotherapy.

DISCOLORATION

Following either sclerotherapy or laser, your treated spider veins commonly appear brown due to breakdown of blood within the veins. Discoloration disappears in 80 percent of women within 6 weeks, 95 percent within 12 weeks, and the remainder within 6 months. In rare cases of persistence, a different laser may be used to treat the dark discoloration.

Avoiding iron supplements for one month before treatment may reduce your risk. Those with dark skin are at higher risk. The lighter your skin, the less likely you are to have dark discoloration, and the more likely you are to have light discoloration.

Light discoloration occurs in 10 percent of women who have spider veins treated with laser. These discolorations become evident within a few weeks and usually improve within a few months. Light discoloration does not occur following sclerotherapy.

SKIN DEATH

If the chemical is injected into skin or fat surrounding your spider veins, rather than the vein itself, it may cause a small area of skin death. This will result in a small open wound. If this occurs, the wound will heal in 5 to 10 days and may leave a small scar. Skin death is not a risk following laser therapy.

SWELLING

Swelling may occur if spider veins around your ankles are injected. Swelling occurs in fewer than 5 percent of those treated, can be prevented by wearing compression hose, and improves within two weeks. Ankle swelling is uncommon following laser therapy.

Cost

Sclerotherapy costs between $100 and $400 per session. Laser treatment costs $400 to $800 per session. Expect to pay more if your spider veins are extensive or if the treatments are performed by a physician rather than a supervised technician.

Duration of Results

Once your treated spider veins are no longer visible, you can anticipate that they will not return. However, in some cases of sclerotherapy, spider veins temporarily disappear only to return within two weeks. This can usually be prevented with the recommended period of compression.

Regardless of treatment, you should anticipate the development of new spider veins over time, just as you would if your spider veins had not been treated. Spider vein therapy treats current spider veins but does not prevent new ones.

Spider Veins on the Face

Spider veins may occur anywhere, but are particularly annoying when they occur on the face. Facial spider veins tend to be red, whereas leg spider veins tend to be blue. Red spider veins are more difficult to eliminate due to their robust circulation. Sclerotherapy of red spider veins has been ineffective and unreliable.

Electrodessication involves burning spider veins with electrical current delivered through a pinpoint device. This technique requires several treatments, poses a risk of scarring, and causes temporary discoloration.

Laser therapy of facial spider veins is the treatment of choice. Laser treatment causes minor bruising, which usually improves within a week. You may need two to four treatments to achieve your desired result. Immediately following treatment, you may apply makeup and will be presentable. However, the mild bruising may be a temporary hindrance.

Tattoos

Tattoos can be considered in two very different ways in cosmetic surgery. First, cosmetic tattoos, which obviate the need for some daily makeup application, can be professionally placed. Alternatively, decorative tattoos that were previously obtained at a parlor can be removed.

Placement of Cosmetic Tattoos

Cosmetic tattooing, or *micropigmentation*, can mimic eyeliner, eyebrow pencil, and lip liner. When placed by a trained medical professional, these makeup tattoos can appear natural and attractive. The greatest advantage of tattooed makeup is not needing to bother with daily application. Also, by the

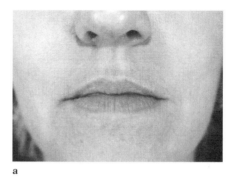

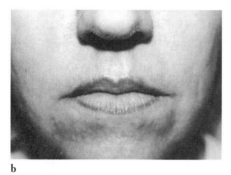
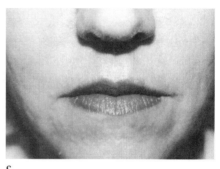

(a) Before placement of permanent lip liner. (b) After placement of permanent lip liner, without lipstick. (c) After placement of permanent lip liner, wearing lipstick.

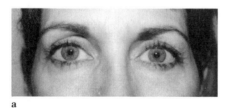
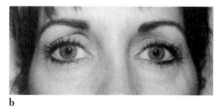

(a) Before placement of permanent eyeliner. (b) After placement of permanent eyeliner.

end of the day, tattooed makeup will not fade. The greatest disadvantage is that it is permanent. So, unless you are certain that it is what you wish, you should not have it.

Cosmetic tattoos are applied in your plastic surgeon's office. A nurse or other trained medical professional will use a tattoo gun to inject permanent ink into your skin. The procedure takes one to two hours. Many find this procedure uncomfortable and choose to have the area numbed prior to tattooing. All tattoos will initially appear brighter or darker than desired, but will fade over several days. When red tattoo pigment is used, such as in lip liner, the tattoo will turn dark brown initially, but will return to the desired color in a few days. Some tattoos also appear crusty for a few days.

The cost of cosmetic tattooing varies depending on the extent of tattooing, the training of the person performing it, and the quality of result. The cost for tattooing a single area, such as the lips, eyes, or eyebrows, ranges from $300 to $1,500.

Beware Nonprofessional Cosmetic Tattooing

Cosmetic tattoos currently are available everywhere and are not closely regulated. Your greatest risk in cosmetic tattooing is having an untrained individual perform this procedure. If they use contaminated needles, infections can be transmitted or the ink may not be of medical quality and may cause irritation.

Cosmetic tattooing of blush on the cheeks is commonly performed by nonprofessionals and often looks distinctly unnatural. Natural cheek color changes from season to season, day to day, and moment to moment. A tattoo does not change and will therefore appear unnatural. If you later regret the decision to have blush tattoos, removal may be difficult, as flesh colored tattoos may turn black in response to laser removal.

If your eyebrow tattoo is placed high, you may have a permanent look of surprise and eyeliner placement has little room for error. If a cosmetic tattoo is botched, removal (with laser) may damage the hair follicles and result in loss of eyelashes or eyebrows. Placement of cosmetic tattoos demands precision.

Do not take cosmetic tattooing lightly. When performed in your plastic surgeon's office you have the greatest chance for a satisfactory outcome. Tattooing outside of your physician's office may be fraught with risk.

> *A woman had lower eyelid liner placed at a beauty parlor. Her tattoo had been injected into fat rather than skin. Because fat cannot retain pigment as skin does, black ink spread throughout her lower eyelid, giving her the appearance of a black eye. Numerous laser treatments performed by another plastic surgeon finally improved her problem.*

> *A woman received a lip liner tattoo at a spa, but it was placed too thick and too high. It gave her the appearance of a fat lip. When she returned to the spa to complain, the aesthetician said she could fix the problem by over-tattooing it in white. Because the white tattoo did not match her skin, it looked like a permanent milk-mustache. Frustrated, this woman sought help from a plastic surgeon, only to discover that white tattoos are among the most difficult to remove and have a risk of turning black in the process.*

Removal of Decorative Tattoos

Many choose to have decorative tattoos in youth but live to regret this decision.

Options for tattoo removal include surgical excision, dermabrasion, and laser. Surgical excision is best employed for small tattoos on loose skin but always leaves a scar. Dermabrasion involves sanding the skin with a rotating wire brush and may leave a scar or a pale area. Even after several treatments, the tattoo may still be visible.

Laser has largely supplanted surgical excision and dermabrasion for the removal of tattoos. Lasers target tattoo ink and rapidly heat it. Heat causes ink to expand and break up into smaller particles. The body is able to then absorb the small ink fragments and carry them away.

Each laser targets a different family of colors. Following each laser session, there will be partial clearing of one family of colors. To completely remove a family of colors, two to four sessions may be required. Because most tattoos are comprised of multiple color families, several lasers may be required. If three lasers are required to remove one tattoo, and each laser must be used three times, a total of nine laser sessions will be necessary. Some tattoos require 15 to 20 laser treatments for complete removal.

Multiple Treatments

Many factors determine the number of treatments necessary. Tattoos obtained in a tattoo parlor are difficult to remove because professional tattoos are typically deep, dark, and made with complex ink. Homemade tattoos are variable in their difficulty of removal based on the type of ink used and the depth they were placed. New tattoos are difficult to remove because they have a higher concentration of ink than old ones. Older tattoos have a lower concentration of ink because as a tattoo ages, the body absorbs some of the ink. Turquoise tattoos are particularly difficult to remove, because no laser effectively targets that color. Red, white, and flesh-colored tattoos are also troublesome (see "Complications").

The total number of treatments necessary cannot be known for sure at the outset. The common range is between 6 and 12. Treatments may be performed every one or two months or may be spaced over several years. The tattoo will begin to fade one week after each treatment and will continue to fade for several months. Some choose to save money by discontinuing treatments before the tattoo is completely removed. Others pursue laser therapy until there are no detectable signs of the tattoo.

Some people choose to over-tattoo to hide an undesirable tattoo. This is especially common when the original tattoo contains the name of a former lover. If you have done this, expect that you will need even more laser treatments.

Complications

Permanent scarring occurs in fewer than 3 percent of those treated. Permanent bleaching or fading of the treated area may occur, particularly after dermabrasion. Bleaching is more common in dark-skinned individuals. Laser removal of red, white, and flesh-colored inks is notoriously difficult. These ink particles may contain iron, which turns black after treatment. It may then be impossible to remove this black pigment. If you have red, white, or flesh colors in your tattoo, your surgeon should test their response by performing laser treatment on a small area before treating the entire tattoo. If it does not turn black, laser treatment of the entire tattoo should be safe.

Cost

The typical cost is $400 to $800 per session. If your tattoo is extensive, expect to pay more. Since 5 to 20 sessions may be required, the total fee may range from $2,000 to $16,000. (This is yet another reason to choose tattoos carefully and think twice before having them applied.)

Unwanted Hair

Women have long tried to rid themselves of unwanted hair of the face, legs, underarms, abdomen, and groin. Waxing, plucking, and electrolysis have all been employed, but are painful and must be repeated regularly. Laser hair removal is the newest treatment option.

The laser causes controlled damage to hair follicles, causing them to go into shock temporarily. While in shock, the follicles do not generate hair.

Duration

Hair will eventually return but will not do so for at least two months in 80 percent of women. Some have enjoyed one or two year periods without hair growth but most require regular treatments at three to four month intervals. When hair returns, it is usually thinner and lighter. Arrested hair growth following six treatments has been reported but should not be expected.

JUDIE, *a 36-year-old investment advisor, had pubic hair that extended to her groins and thighs. Because she spent her summers in a bathing suit, she made many attempts at hair removal. Waxing and electrolysis were painful. Shaving caused ingrown hairs. Laser hair removal was like a miracle treatment. Each session took about 30 minutes, and hair did not return for three months. Even though she needs repeat treatments, she is happier than she was with waxing, shaving, and electrolysis.*

What to Expect

Treatments are performed in your doctor's office by a nurse or a trained technician and last from 15 to 90 minutes depending on the size of area treated. You may return to work immediately after treatment. Unlike waxing, you may shave immediately prior to your laser hair removal. Anticipate that your treated skin may turn pale purple, and this will persist for several days. Some areas may scab and blister temporarily.

Recovery

As with all laser therapies, avoid unprotected sun for three to six months afterward to prevent sunburn and dark discoloration. You may also develop light spots on your treated areas. Both problems usually normalize within a few weeks. Wearing sunscreen with a sun protection factor (SPF) of 15 or higher will help protect you from dark discoloration. (If you like to tan, note that quarterly or biannual treatments will prohibit tanning year-round.)

Cost

Cost ranges from $300 to $1,000 per session, with a typical fee of $600. If you have extensive hair growth on your back, abdomen, and thighs, expect to pay more.

Laser Hair Removal Is Not Permanent

Laser hair removal has never been proved to be permanent. Advertising laws, however, allow the providers of laser hair removal to claim that it is permanent if it lasts for at least three months. Do not be deceived. Laser hair removal is not permanent.

However, laser technology is evolving. A laser that reliably and permanently removes hair may be available in the future.

ELIZABETH, *a 67-year-old retired schoolteacher, had recovered from a facelift, eyelid surgery, and forehead lift. She was pleased with her results but thought her thin lips were "a giveaway" that she was actually older than she appeared. Lip augmentation gave her full youthful lips and restored harmony to her face.*

Thin Lips

Full lips are a sign of youth and sensuality, whereas thin lips can reveal true age and detract from an otherwise youthful appearance.

Although all women's lips thin as they age, some young women have thin lips also. Thus, women of all ages seek lip augmentation.

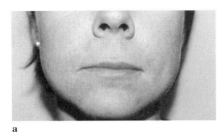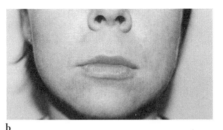

a   b

(a) Before lip augmentation. (b) After lip augmentation with Alloderm.

Augmentation may be performed for one or both lips. Most women choose to have both lips augmented to preserve harmony.

Augmentation Options

Available materials for lip augmentation can be classified as liquid form or sheet form.

Liquid Form

Liquid injections were once the mainstay of lip augmentation, but they lost favor due to short-lived effects. They contain collagen or fat (see Chapter 11). Unfortunate experience has shown that liquid silicone should never be used.

Sheet Form

The most common type of lip augmentation is in sheet form. The three options for this are Alloderm, fascia, or Gore-Tex. (These materials are also sometimes used to fill creases around the mouth.)

ALLODERM

Alloderm is freeze-dried collagen that is prepared in sheet form. It is obtained from deceased human donors. (See "Obtaining Tissues from Deceased Human Donors," Chapter 6.) Cadaver skin can be processed into thin pliable sheets that can be rolled and placed through tiny incisions to fill the entire lip. The incisions are in the corner of the mouth and heal imperceptibly.

Beware Liquid Silicone Injections

If your doctor suggests liquid silicone injection, under no circumstances should you agree. Instead, report that physician to the state medical board. Liquid silicone (which differs from contained silicone gel breast implants) was injected into the faces and breasts of numerous women during the 1960s and 1970s. The initial results were aesthetic, soft, and natural. However, within weeks, months, or years, the injected areas became hard, lumpy, red, and painful. Some women appeared unnatural, unsightly, and even diseased. Because silicone disseminated throughout the injected area, its removal was not a simple procedure. Unfortunately, some doctors still perform liquid silicone injections.

Swelling and bruising improve in one week. Your lips will feel stiff for four weeks, and you will have difficulty puckering during this time. The final result is soft, natural, and pliable. Alloderm placement, unlike liquid collagen injections, need only be performed once to achieve the desired result.

Alloderm may partially or completely reabsorb, especially if placed too deeply. Regardless of where it is placed, expect some degree of shrinkage during the first year. Transmission of infection from the human donor, a theoretical risk, has never occurred.

The cost of Alloderm is $500 for a piece large enough to augment both lips. Your surgeon will charge an additional $1,000–$2,000 to place implants in both lips. Due to its ease of placement and consistent results, Alloderm is becoming the lip implant material of choice for many plastic surgeons. Be aware, however, that Alloderm lip augmentation has been performed widely since only the mid 1990s. Long-term results will not be known for at least two decades.

Creases Around the Mouth

Creases around the mouth, or nasolabial folds, are formed by sagging skin. As mentioned in both Chapters 2 and 11, skin fold wrinkles in this area are best treated with a face-lift. (A face-lift, instead of just camouflaging the creases, addresses their cause.)

Some plastic surgeons offer to fill facial creases as an alternative to face-lift. They use Alloderm or Gore-Tex as an implant material. The same principles and methods explained for lip augmentation pertain to creases around the mouth. Facial soft-tissue augmentation is less of a procedure than a face-lift, but provides less improvement. But results have been variable in effect and duration. If a face-lift is truly needed, do not expect much from an implant.

FASCIA

Fascia is dense, white connective tissue that envelops your muscles. In many areas of the body, fascia is unnecessary and can be harvested for cosmetic use. One such area is the temporoparietal fascia, called *TP fascia*, which is a layer of your scalp above either ear. TP fascia can be harvested through a small incision that heals inconspicuously because it is hidden behind the hairline.

TP fascia offers the advantage of using your own tissue. The theoretic risk of transmission of infection does not exist. (Of course, as with any operation, infection from the environment may occur, but this, too, may be lower with use of your own tissue.) Extrusion is also unlikely.

But TP fascia requires surgery for harvest, hence another area of discomfort and potential complications. Also, it will shrink and become absorbed by your body over time. You may eventually seek another lip augmentation.

The cost of this procedure is similar to that of Alloderm placement. You will not have to pay for an implant, but some surgeons may charge more for harvesting your fascia.

GORE-TEX

Gore-Tex is a cross between cloth and rubber and can be used to make implants. If you have Gore-Tex placed but later desire its removal, surgery will be necessary. Gore-Tex may be slightly stiff, but most recipients become accustomed to this. Many surgeons choose to avoid using Gore-Tex because of their concern that it may extrude or become infected as with any synthetic implant. If it is placed deeply and away from the incision, extrusion and infection are unlikely. One advantage over Alloderm is that Gore-Tex will never shrink and will always maintain its size. The cost of Gore-Tex is $500 to augment both lips. Surgeon's fee is an additional $1,000 to $2,000.

What to Expect

Lip augmentation is an office procedure and is usually performed under local anesthesia. If injected materials are used, such as liquid collagen or fat, incisions are not needed. Instead your surgeon uses a small needle to fill out your lips. If sheets of material are used, your surgeon will make small incisions at the corners of your mouth. The sheets of material will then be threaded through your lips to provide smooth, even augmentation. The incisions will become invisible within two weeks (fig. 13-2).

Recovery

You may return to your regular routine immediately, unless you were sedated. If you were sedated, then you may resume your usual activities the following day. Swelling and bruising last for three days to two weeks. Discomfort is minimal, and prescription pain medication is often not required.

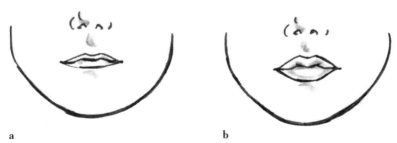

a   b

FIGURE 13-2 *Lip augmentation. (a) Thin lips before augmentation. (b) Full lips following augmentation. Scars are not shown because typically, they are not visible.*

Complications

Lip augmentation is a relatively simple procedure with few problems. However, as with all surgical procedures, complications may occur.

Cold Sore Outbreak

Cold sores are viral outbreaks, usually on the lips. Although they may occur during a cold, they are not due to the cold virus. When there are no sores, the virus that causes them lies dormant. If your body becomes stressed (during illness, emotional stress, physical trauma, or surgery), the dormant virus may awaken and trigger cold sores.

The presence of active cold sores at the time of your procedure may cause a severe outbreak afterward. The outbreak will not be limited to your lips; it may involve your entire face. Such an outbreak may leave you with unsightly scars. If you have active cold sores, your surgeon will probably recommend postponing the procedure until after they have healed. Even if you have no active cold sores, your surgeon will probably treat you with antiviral medication as a precaution.

Extrusion

Implants that are placed in sheet form, such as Alloderm, fascia, or Gore-Tex, may work their way out through one of the incisions. To prevent this uncommon and unpleasant complication, your surgeon will aim to keep the implant away from the healing incision. If extrusion does occur, your surgeon will probably remove the implant, allow your lips to heal, and later augment your lips with a material that is less likely to extrude.

Extrusion following placement of injected material is extremely rare.

Infection

Implants that are placed in sheet form may become infected. You may require antibiotics, removal of the infected implant, or both. If removal is necessary, another implant may be placed six months later, but this procedure may be confounded by scarring. Risk of infection following placement of sheet implants is less than 1 percent. Risk of infection following injection is even less common.

Reabsorption

Implants made of collagen, fat, or fascia will be absorbed by varying degrees. Some are completely absorbed over time. Gore-Tex will never shrink or become absorbed.

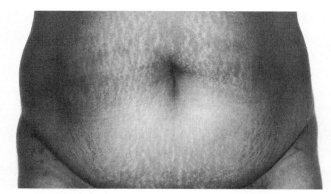

Stretch marks.

Stretch Marks

During periods of rapid weight gain, skin will stretch to accommodate increased body volume. Because skin is elastic, it will tolerate significant stretching over a short period of time, such as during pregnancy. At some point, however, the skin will reach a limit, and the deepest layer will tear instead of stretching further. When the deep layer tears, the overlying skin remains intact but appears thin and streaky. These streaks are called *stretch marks*. Once stretch marks occur, they are permanent.

Although some physicians claim that lasers improve stretch marks, there is no scientific evidence to support this. Most plastic surgeons think that lasers are ineffective in treating this problem. (Lasers are effective in removing, vaporizing, and breaking down tissues. They do not generally repair tissues. Stretch marks represent torn tissue. Hence, improvement should not be expected from laser treatment.)

Laser technology is evolving, so there may someday be a laser that is effective for stretch marks. In the meantime, beware. Stretch mark removal is an arena in which false claims prevail.

Abdominal stretch marks occur primarily below the belly button. Because much of the skin below the belly button is removed during a tummy tuck, stretch marks in this area are also removed. If you have stretch marks below your belly button, you may wish to be evaluated for a tummy tuck (see Chapter 9). There is no other proved treatment for stretch marks.

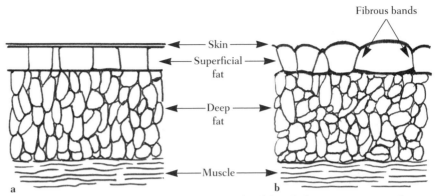

FIGURE 13-3 *Cross-section of the skin. (a) Superficial and deep fat layers in someone without cellulite. (b) The superficial layer of fat become distended, causing the fat to bulge around the skin-tethering bands. This creates the dimpled appearance of cellulite.*

Cellulite

Cellulite is a common but unattractive dimpling and puckering of skin. Cellulite is caused by a combination of fibrous bands and superficial fat. In areas such as the buttocks and thighs, inelastic fibrous bands connect the skin and the deep layer of fat, passing through the superficial layer of fat. When superficial fat compartments become distended with fat, dimpling shows where the fibrous bands tether the skin (fig. 13-3).

Currently no absolute treatment for cellulite exists, but some have found improvement through outer thigh and buttock lift (see Chapter 9). (Some physicians have advertised that their lasers can treat cellulite. Do not be deceived by these ads, as no such treatments are considered effective at this time.)

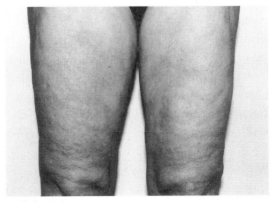

Cellulite.

Endermologie

Endermologie is a nonsurgical procedure that theoretically stimulates break-down of fat and cellulite. In it, a technician uses a machine to apply gentle pressure and suction to your skin. The machine looks and sounds somewhat like a handheld vacuum cleaner and its application feels similar to a deep massage. Sessions last 40 minutes and are conducted one to two times per week until a point of diminishing improvement is reached. Those who gain benefit begin to see results within 10 sessions and plateau between the 15th and 20th session. Thereafter, monthly sessions are required to maintain the result.

Advantages

Endermologie is generally affordable. Each treatment costs $80 to $100. The average cost to achieve plateau is between $1,200 and $2,000. Maintenance is then $80 to $100 per month. There is no pain and no recovery time. In addition to improved body contour, you may see an improvement in cellulite and skin tone.

Disadvantages

Even though the price seems low compared to liposuction, the final outcome depends on several factors and is not guaranteed. One key factor is the skill of the technician who performs the procedure. Another important factor is diet and exercise, which is necessary to achieve a benefit from endermologie. Body metabolism must be geared toward fat breakdown in order for ender-mologie to be effective. If a diet and exercise regime is not followed, little improvement will result. Women who cannot commit to regular treatments, diet, and exercise should not pursue endermologie.

Monthly maintenance sessions can be costly at $1,200 per year, particu-larly when considering that your results will not last. Within three to five years, you will return to your pre-endermologie state despite strict adherence to maintenance sessions, diet, and exercise. You must then resume weekly sessions to re-achieve your previous plateau.

Pregnant women and those with varicose veins are not candidates for endermologie. Varicose veins may burst if treated with endermologie.

Other Applications

Endermologie may be used with liposuction. Some surgeons perform ender-mologie in the operating room immediately prior to liposuction. They think it softens fat, aids suctioning, and smooths the final result. Other surgeons ask their patients to have endermologie sessions following liposuction, once discomfort resolves. Endermologie may optimize the result of liposuction by smoothing fat and stimulating skin retraction. Although clinical experience supports these uses for endermologie, proof of benefit is lacking.

Questions to Ask Your Plastic Surgeon

Can laser solve my problem?

Will the effects be temporary or permanent?

How many laser treatments will I need?

What materials do you recommend for lip augmentation?

How long will my lip augmentation last?

Controversy

Many plastic surgeons feel that the results seen through endermologie are no better than the results of diet and exercise alone. Lack of studies explaining why endermologie works and proving its effectiveness contributes to skepticism. Other surgeons are convinced that diet and exercise alone cannot account for the changes they have seen. Clearly, plastic surgeons have not reached a consensus on endermologie.

Concluding Thoughts

The currently available treatments for minor skin problems can be relatively safe, effective, convenient, and

Tips and Traps

Laser treatment is not a panacea.

Varicose veins must be treated before spider veins.

Injections are most effective for medium to large spider veins; laser is most effective for small to medium spider veins.

A supervised technician may safely perform laser spider vein treatment, laser hair removal, laser tattoo removal, and laser treatments for minor skin discoloration. A physician must perform laser treatment for wrinkles.

Beware of laypeople who offer cosmetic tattooing of your face.

Laser hair removal offers many benefits, but it is not permanent.

Understand that Alloderm, fascia, and Gore-Tex offer different advantages. No single implant material is right for every woman.

Ask for antiviral prophylaxis prior to lip surgery, even if you do not recall ever having a cold sore.

Expect difficulty puckering for a month following Alloderm placement in your lips.

Seek both upper and lower lip augmentations to maintain harmony.

Laser is not effective in removing stretch marks.

Plastic surgeons are divided over whether or not endermologie offers a true benefit.

affordable. They may impose little recovery time, but they are not without risk. For example, any time you allow placement of an implant in your body, you are opening the door to potential complications. Be certain that you are fully informed before having any procedure, no matter how innocuous it may seem.

Afterword

You have numerous questions, some of which have been answered by this book; others of which have been sparked. Among the many answers you are seeking, one stands out above all others, regardless of who you are or which procedure you seek: "Will cosmetic surgery be worth it?"

In the beginning, you will ask, "Will this be worth the time, expense, potential risks, and cost?" You will understandably be uncertain. In the end, you will ask, "Was it worth it?" You will more easily answer the latter question, because you will have gone through the experience of surgery, seen your result, and (hopefully) emerged complication free. There will be few unknowns.

Although only you can make your decision, it may help you to know the experience of others. As millions have gone before you, what did they conclude?*

About 95 percent of those who have undergone cosmetic surgery were very satisfied. It is no wonder, therefore, that 58 percent of those undergoing cosmetic surgery seek multiple procedures or return at a later date for additional surgery. It is also no surprise that cosmetic surgery nearly doubled in popularity every four years during the 1990s.

Temper this with the knowledge that 5 percent were dissatisfied with their choice to have cosmetic surgery. Some were even devastated. If they were

*The following statistics are for patients of surgeons certified by the American Board of Plastic Surgery. It does not include statistics from the patients of other physicians.

277

able to turn back the clock, they would not have had it. So, how can you get yourself out of the 5 percent and into the 95 percent?

You can minimize the risk of dissatisfaction by identifying and consulting with a qualified plastic surgeon. Visualize your expectations and carefully discuss them with your surgeon. You may try to safeguard yourself from disappointment, but be forewarned that there is no foolproof way. Emotions sway the intellect and alter the perception of reality.

You can reduce your risk of complications by complying with the instructions of your surgeon. But you can never eliminate risk, and the more you understand and accept potential complications, the better you will deal with them if they arise.

The popularity of cosmetic surgery speaks for itself. Yet, in the end, the decision is yours alone. This book and your plastic surgeon can provide you only with information and expertise. The rest is up to you.

Appendix

Summary Table for All Procedures

	GREATEST ADVANTAGES	GREATEST DISADVANTAGES	RECOVERY[1]	COST[2]
Face-lift	Improves heavy cheeks, jowls, and loose skin of the face and neck	Does not improve skin quality; does not affect forehead or eyelids	10–14 days	$8,000
Forehead lift	Improves forehead wrinkles, scowl lines, and droopy eyebrows	Does not tighten loose eyelid skin	7–14 days	$4,000
Eyelid surgery	Improves eyelid bagginess and puffiness	Does not improve crow's feet or eyebrows	3–14 days	$4,500
Nose surgery	Can change nasal appearance in numerous ways	20% of patients need revision surgery	1–2 weeks	$5,000
Chin or cheek implant	Provides stronger facial contour and profile	All synthetic implants pose potential risks	1–2 weeks	$3,500
Lip augmentation	Can create full lips	Depending on the material used, the results may be temporary	3–14 days	$2,000
Breast augmentation	Can enlarge breasts to desired size	All synthetic implants pose potential risks	3–10 days	$6,000
Breast lift	Can raise breasts to a more youthful position	Scars can be extensive	3–7 days	$5,300

	GREATEST ADVANTAGES	GREATEST DISADVANTAGES	RECOVERY[1]	COST[2]
Tummy tuck	Can restore a flat, tight abdomen	Surgery is much more extensive than the name implies	1–2 weeks	$6,500
Inner thigh lift	Will tighten loose inner thigh skin; scars are hidden	Moderately large operation	1–2 weeks	$5,000
Outer thigh and buttock lift	Will lift droopy outer thighs and buttocks; may improve cellulite in some	Recovery and scars are extensive	1–3 weeks	$6,500
Total body lift	See tummy tuck, inner thigh lift, outer thigh/buttock lift	Surgery, recovery, and scars are extensive	3–6 weeks	$14,500
Liposuction	Will reduce localized areas of fat deposit	Will not tighten loose skin; will not improve cellulite	5–14 days	Variable
Skin care	Improves skin color, tone, texture, and complexion	Final results not seen until after 6–12 months of regular use; will not affect dynamic wrinkles	Immediate	$30–50 per month
Micro peel	Improves skin color, tone, texture, and complexion within several weeks	Multiple peels and maintenance peels required; will not affect dynamic wrinkles	Immediate	$60–80 per peel
Superficial peel	Dramatic improvement in skin color, tone, texture, and complexion within several weeks	3 days of dry, flaky skin after each peel; will not affect dynamic wrinkles	Immediate	$80–120 per peel
Medium peel	Dramatic improvement in skin color, tone, texture, and complexion within a week, improves fine wrinkles	5 days of obvious flaking afterward; several peels may be necessary; minimal effect on dynamic wrinkles	4–7 days	$2,000 for full face
Deep peel	Overwhelming and lasting effect on wrinkles	Unnaturally pale complexion is permanent	10–14 days	$4,000 full face
Erbium laser	Improves dynamic wrinkles, fine wrinkles, and acne scars	Not as effective as carbon dioxide laser	4–7 days	$3,400 full face
Carbon dioxide laser	Improves dynamic wrinkles, fine wrinkles, and acne scars; may be more effective than erbium	Lengthy recovery	10–14 days	$4,200 for full face

	GREATEST ADVANTAGES	GREATEST DISADVANTAGES	RECOVERY[1]	COST[2]
Derma-brasion	*Improves acne scars and lip wrinkles*	*Risk of light discoloration; need for multiple treatments*	*7–10 days*	*$4,000 full face*
Collagen injection	*Provides temporary improvement of deeply creased wrinkles*	*Requires multiple treatments necessary*	*Immediate*	*$500–$1500 each*
Botox injection	*Dramatic improvement in dynamic wrinkles*	*Must be repeated every 3–6 months*	*Immediate*	*$1,000*
Laser treatment of spider veins	*Most effective for small to medium spider veins*	*Causes temporary brown discoloration, usually three sessions are required*	*Immediate*	*$600 per treatment*
Injection of spider veins	*Most effective for medium or large spider veins*	*Requires up to 6 sessions; may not clear all spider veins*	*Immediate*	*$250 per treatment*
Cosmetic lip liner or eyeliner tattoo	*Obviates the need for daily makeup placement*	*If not performed by a skilled professional, it may yield disastrous results*	*Immediate*	*$800*
Laser removal of decorative tattoos	*Results in gradual disappearance of tattoo without scars*	*Requires multiple treatments*	*Immediate*	*$600 per treatment*
Laser hair removal	*Arrests hair growth for 2–4 months, when hair returns it is lighter and thinner*	*Is not permanent; requires quarterly treatments*	*Immediate*	*$800 per treatment*
Laser stretch mark removal	*None*	*There is no evidence that laser improves stretch marks*	*Immediate*	*Irrelevant*
Endermologie	*May improve cellulite and tighten skin*	*Benefits are unproved, temporary, and rely upon regular treatments*	*Immediate*	*$90 per treatment*

[1]*"Recovery" is the time required before one can resume sedentary work and be comfortable in public either with makeup or with the treated part covered.*

[2]*"Cost" is the average cost across the United States in the year 2000 and includes surgeon fee, operating room fee, anesthesia fee, and implant fee, where relevant. (Add 2 percent per year to arrive at the average cost after the year 2000.) The cost of each procedure in or around New York is about 50 percent higher than the rest of the country. If you are having more than one procedure, reduce the total by 10 percent. When multiple treatments are customary, the cost listed is per treatment.*

Glossary

Abdominoplasty: *Same as* Tummy tuck.

Adrenaline: *Same as* Epinephrine.

Aesthetic surgery: *Same as* Cosmetic surgery.

AHA: *Same as* Alpha hydroxy acids.

Alloderm: Freeze-dried collagen that is obtained from deceased human donors and prepared in sheet form for soft-tissue augmentation.

Alpha hydroxy acids (AHAs): Naturally occurring fruit acids that stimulate growth and turnover of skin cells, improve skin texture, reduce fine wrinkles, and restore skin vitality. The AHAs include glycolic acid, citric acid, malic acid, and lactic acid.

American Board of Plastic Surgery (ABPS): The only board recognized by the American Board of Medical Specialties for certifying plastic surgeons in the United States.

American Society of Plastic and Reconstructive Surgeons (ASPRS): The predominant organization in plastic surgery, which inducts only surgeons who are certified by the American Board of Plastic Surgery. 800-635-0635, www.plasticsurgery.org.

Anatomic breast implant: A breast implant that is teardrop shaped rather than round.

Anesthesia: *See* local anesthesia, sedation anesthesia, or general anesthesia.

Anesthesiologist: Medical doctor who specializes in making surgery safe and comfortable via medications.

Anesthesiologist's fee: Usually depends on the length of the procedure. (If your surgeon administers your sedation, or if only local anesthesia is used, there should be no anesthesiologist's fee.)

Areola: Pigmented area around the breast nipple.

Attached earlobe: Also called pixie ear. Undesirable appearance of the earlobe following face-lift. When too much skin has been removed near the earlobe, the earlobe is pulled downward and appears to attach to the surrounding skin, rather than hang independently.

Augmentation mammoplasty: *Same as* Breast augmentation.

Autologen: Collagen from your own skin, harvested during a previous operation and processed into liquid form for injection.

Autologous fat graft: Fat obtained through liposuction for injection into another part of the body.

Beta hydroxy acids (BHAs): Chemicals with slightly more potency than alpha hydroxy acids. Often used for superficial peels. Example: salicylic acid.

BHA: *Same as* Beta hydroxy acid.

Bleaching agents: Improve or prevent dark discoloration by suppressing the activity of pigment-producing cells.

Blepharoplasty: *Same as* Eyelid surgery.

Body contouring: Any procedure that reshapes the body, such as liposuction, tummy tuck, or thigh lift.

Botox: Medical-grade botulism toxin. Weakens the muscles responsible for dynamic wrinkles, causing the wrinkles to temporarily improve or disappear.

Botulinum toxin: *Same as* Botox.

Bovine collagen: A protein matrix extracted from cow skin, then purified, sterilized, and processed into liquid form for injection into wrinkles.

Breast augmentation: The placement of implants into women with normal breasts that are smaller than desired. One of the three most common cosmetic procedures performed in the United States.

Breast droop: Defined by plastic surgeons based on the position of the nipple compared to the breast crease: *mild* droop exists when the nipple is at the level of the crease, *moderate* droop exists when the nipple is below the crease, and *advanced* droop exists when the nipple is on the lowest part of the breast, pointing downward.

Breast lift: An operation to raise the breast by tightening the skin envelope around it.

Breast ptosis (pronounced *toe-sis*): Breast droop.

Breast reconstruction: An operation performed on women who have had mastectomies. Restores breast volume and shape, usually to match the other breast. May involve implants or soft-tissue reconstruction, such as a TRAM flap.

Brow lift: *Same as* Forehead lift.

Buttock lift: *Same as* Outer thigh and buttock lift.

Buttock/outer thigh lift: *Same as* Outer thigh and buttock lift.

Button chin: Unnaturally small or round chin, which may result if a chin implant is too small or narrow.

Cadaver bone: Human bone, harvested from donors shortly after death.

Cannula: *Same as* Liposuction rod.

Canthopexy: Surgical procedure to tighten and raise the lower eyelid.

Capsular contractures: Abnormally tight scars that may form around a breast implant. *Mild* contractures cause the breast to feel slightly firm and the implant edges to be felt through the skin. *Moderate* contractures cause the breast to feel firm and the implant to be both felt and perceived visually through the skin. *Severe* contractures cause the breast to feel hard, distorted, and painful.

Cauterization: Use of low-level electrical current on tiny blood vessels during surgery to stop them from bleeding.

Cellulite: A common but unattractive dimpling and puckering of the skin. Due to combination of superficial fat, fibrous tissue, and gravity.

Cerebrospinal fluid: Natural body fluid that bathes the brain and spinal cord. May be called "CSF" by physicians or "brain fluid" by laypeople.

Cheek augmentation: An operation to increase the cheeks' projection via placement of an implant.

Cheek lift: Also called mid-face-lift. A limited version of the subperiosteal face-lift. Effective in rejuvenating the cheek area.

Chin augmentation: Also called mentoplasty. An operation to increase the chin's projection via placement of an implant.

Citric acid: An alpha hydroxy acid (AHA). Derived from oranges and grapefruits.

Collagen: The protein matrix of the skin. Sometimes called the meat of the skin. May be obtained from cow skin, cadaver skin, or your own skin—refined, sterilized, and processed for safe use. So far, there are four main types of collagen for cosmetic injection: bovine collagen, Autologen, Isolagen, and Dermalogen.

Computer imaging: A technology that enables surgeons to take your photograph and manipulate it to show you how you might look following your proposed procedure. May inflate expectations.

Connective Tissue Diseases (CTDs): Autoimmune diseases—the body's own defense system identifies normal body tissue as foreign and so attacks it. Joints become stiff, skin develops rashes, muscles ache, and the body tires easily. Examples of CTDs include rheumatoid arthritis, lupus, scleroderma, fibromyalgia, and chronic fatigue syndrome.

Cornea: Outer layer of the pupil.

Corneal abrasion: Inadvertent scratch to the cornea. Temporarily painful. Treated by patching the eye closed for one to three days.

Corrugators: Muscles that, together with the procerus muscles, are responsible for vertical frown lines between the eyebrows.

Cosmetic plastic surgery: *Same as* Cosmetic surgery.

Cosmetic surgery: Surgery that focuses solely on improving appearance. A subspecialty of plastic surgery.

Cosmetic tattooing: Permanent tattooing that mimics eyeliner, eyebrow pencil, or lip liner.

Cost: *Same as* Fees.

Crepe paper wrinkles: Fine wrinkles that occur on the cheeks, where sun exposure is high and the skin is relatively thin.

Crow's feet: Wrinkles that radiate from the corners of the eyes. Especially prominent while smiling or squinting.

Dark circles: Dark areas of the lower eyelids that give a tired appearance. May be caused by shadows or discolored skin.

Dark discoloration: Dark, blotchy, irregular patches of skin, typically on the face or neck. May develop following laser treatment, chemical peel, or pregnancy.

Deep chemical peel: Procedure whereby a chemical, usually phenol, is applied to the skin, causing a controlled injury. The most effective chemical peel in treating wrinkles, which are markedly improved and in many cases eliminated. Leaves the skin permanently pale.

Deep peel: *Same as* Deep chemical peel.

Deep vein thrombosis (DVT): Blood clot, usually within a thigh vein, which may form during or after surgery. Can travel through your bloodstream and lodge in your lungs. Can create catastrophic breathing problems and debilitating leg problems.

Deflation: Complication of saline implants in which the implant leaks and flattens. The body then naturally absorbs the saline.

Dermabrasion: Removal of superficial skin by a process similar to sanding. Allows healthier skin to surface and results in smoother texture and tighter skin.

Dermalogen: Collagen from human cadaver skin that has been sterilized, purified, and processed into liquid form for injection.

Discoloration: *See* Light discoloration, Dark discoloration, or Melasma.

Dog ears: Areas of puckered skin. May occur when there is more skin on one side of an incision than the other. Occurs most commonly when skin is removed as part of a procedure such as tummy tuck.

Droopy upper eyelids: Eyelids that appear to hang at "half-mast." The lower edge of the upper eyelid blocks more than the very top of the iris. Also called *eyelid ptosis.*

Dry eye syndrome: Complication of eyelid surgery in which the eyes feel dry, gritty, and as though there is sand in them. Eyes are actually watery. Vision may be blurred.

Dynamic wrinkles: The result of repetitive facial expressions. Smiling, laughing, frowning, or brooding causes the skin to be moved in the same way over and over again. Each time the skin moves, it creases, eventually forming wrinkles.

Early relapse: Premature return of sagging parts after surgery, well before expected. May occur after face-lift, forehead lift, breast lift, and body lift.

Ectropion: *Same as* Lower eyelid retraction.

Endermologie: A nonsurgical procedure that theoretically stimulates breakdown of fat and cellulite.

Endoscope: Long, thin metal rod with a fiber-optic camera at the tip.

Endoscopic surgery: Uses an endoscope, which is slipped under the skin. Has been applied to forehead lift, breast augmentation, tummy tuck, and face-lift. Allows smaller incisions and hence smaller scars.

Epidermis: Outermost layer of skin.

Epinephrine: Also called adrenaline. Hormone used with local anesthetic to constrict blood vessels and reduce bleeding.

Excise: To surgically remove something, such as a mole or excess skin.

Excision: The act of excising.

Exfoliation: Removal of dead superficial skin cells. Facilitates penetration of stimulants such as alpha hydroxy acid and retin-A.

External ultrasound–assisted liposuction (EUAL): Delivery of ultrasonic energy to skin overlying the fat before performing liposuction.

Extrusion: Erosion of skin or mucosa overlying an implant, which may then become exposed and will likely need to be removed. Extrusion may occur following placement of any implant.

Eyelid ptosis (pronounced *toe-sis*): *Same as* Droopy upper eyelids.

Eyelid surgery: Among the three most commonly performed cosmetic procedures in the United States. May remove excess upper eyelid skin, upper eyelid fat, lower eyelid skin, and lower eyelid fat. May include upper eyelid lift, lower eyelid tightening (canthopexy), or ethnic modification.

Face-lift: Operation to remove excess face and neck skin, while lifting and tightening the remaining skin and tissues.

Facialplasty: *Same as* Face-lift.

Facility fee: Cost charged by the surgery center, hospital, or doctor's office where surgery is to be performed.

Fascia: Dense white connective tissue that envelops your muscles. In some areas of the body, fascia is unnecessary and can be harvested for cosmetic use. In other areas, such as the abdomen, fascia is an important structural element that helps determine body shape.

Fat embolus: Fat globules that migrate into the bloodstream and clump into a larger mass of fat. Can interfere with exchange of oxygen and carbon dioxide if it travels into the lungs. Severe and potentially fatal respiratory problems may result.

Fees: Cosmetic surgery involves fees for the surgeon anesthesiologist facility hospital, and implant. Not all fees apply in every case.

Forehead lift: An operation to raise brow position, reduce lateral hoods, and soften horizontal forehead wrinkles and scowl lines.

Foreheadplasty: *Same as* Forehead lift.

Frontalis muscle: The forehead muscle that raises the eyebrows and causes horizontal forehead wrinkles.

Frown lines: *See* Dynamic wrinkles.

General anesthesia: Induces a deep sleep and temporarily paralyzes the body. Spontaneous breathing stops, so the anesthesiologist places a tube (connected to a respirator) into the windpipe.

Genioplasty: Augmenting the chin by surgically breaking a portion of the chin bone, moving it forward, and securing it with screws or wires.

Glycolic acid: The alpha hydroxy acid (AHA) most commonly used in cosmetic surgery. Derived from sugar cane.

Gore-Tex: A cross between cloth and rubber that is used for implants. Technical name is expanded polytetrafluoroethylene (EPTFE).

Graft: Living tissue, such as fat, cartilage, skin, or bone, that is moved from one part of the body to another. Must receive nourishment from the surrounding tissues.

Grave's disease: Thyroid condition that causes the eyes to bulge outward and the eyelids to appear puffy.

Hematoma: Accumulation of blood within the surgical site after the skin incision has been closed. May require immediate surgery.

Hospital fee: What the hospital charges if you stay overnight following your procedure.

Hydroquinone: A bleaching agent.

Hydroxyapatite: A porous, ceramic material used for facial implants. Resembles sea coral.

Hyperpigmentation: *See* Dark discoloration.

Hypopigmentation: *See* Light discoloration.

Implant deflation: *Same as* Deflation.

Implant extrusion: *Same as* Extrusion.

Implant fee: The cost of medical materials such as breast implants, facial implants, and collagen.

Inframammary crease: The skin crease beneath the breast.

Inner girdle: Fascia of the abdomen.

Inner thigh lift: Removes excess skin from the inner thighs, tightening and lifting the remaining skin.

Iris: The colored ring around the pupil of the eye.

Isolagen: Collagen from your own skin, cloned in a laboratory and processed into liquid form for injection.

Lactic acid: An alpha hydroxy acid (AHA) derived from milk.

Lagophthalmos: *Same as* Upper eyelid retraction.

Lasabrasion: *Same as* Laser resurfacing.

Laser desurfacing: *Same as* Laser resurfacing.

Laser: A tool that emits an intense, focused beam of light. Used to treat wrinkles, scars, birthmarks, spider veins, skin discolorations, age spots, and tattoos.

Laser peeling: *Same as* Laser resurfacing.

Laser resurfacing: Treatment of skin with carbon dioxide laser or erbium laser, which vaporizes the top layers of skin. (Deeper, healthier cells replace the outer damaged cells and allow reorganization, resulting in reduced wrinkles and improved skin tone.)

Laser vaporization: *Same as* Laser resurfacing.

Lateral hoods: Folds of skin between the eyebrow and the eyelid near the outside corner of the eye. Named for the hooded look they give to the eyes.

Lateral thigh and buttock lift: *Same as* Outer thigh and buttock lift.

Lidocaine: A local anesthetic, similar to novocaine.

Light chemical peel: *Same as* Superficial chemical peel.

Light discoloration: Blotchy, irregular patches of skin that are lighter than nearby skin. May develop within several weeks of laser treatment or dermabrasion.

Lipoplasty: *Same as* Liposuction.

Liposculpture: *Same as* Liposuction.

Liposuction: The most popular cosmetic procedure performed in the United States. Removes local fat deposits. The three methods of liposuction are traditional, ultrasonic, and external ultrasound–assisted.

Liposuction cannulas: *Same as* Liposuction rods.

Liposuction garments: Similar to a girdle. Essential for good results following liposuction. Provides firm pressure and support to suctioned areas. Facilitates skin retraction and optimizes final body contour.

Liposuction rods: Long, thin, metal rods used to suction fat during liposuction.

Liquid silicone: A substance that was injected into breasts and lips for augmentation. Distorted and hardened the tissue; no longer used.

Local anesthesia: Injection of local anesthetic agents only. No sedation, paralysis, or deep sleep. (When doctors refer to performing a procedure "under local," this is what they mean.)

Local anesthetic: Medications such as lidocaine that are injected into an area of the body to cause temporary numbness there. Similar to novocaine. Some wear off within a few hours, others last for half a day. Used both in local anesthesia and sedation anesthesia.

Love handles: Fat deposits above the hip bones. "Hips."

Lower body lift: *Same as* Total body lift.

Lower lid retraction: A complication of eyelid surgery. The lower lid is pulled downward, due either to a loose lower eyelid or removal of too much skin.

Malar implants: Cheek implants.

Malic acid: An alpha hydroxy acid (AHA) derived from apples.

Mammogram: Breast x-ray.

Mammography: *See* Mammogram.

Marionette lines: Vertical creases from the corners of the mouth to the jowls.

Mastectomy: Surgical removal of a breast, usually for cancer.

Mastopexy: *Same as* Breast lift.

Matting: The sudden appearance of new spider veins. May occur anywhere on an extremity recently treated with sclerotherapy or laser for spider veins.

Medial thigh lift: *Same as* Inner thigh lift.

Medium chemical peel: A controlled injury to the skin from applying a chemical, usually TCA in order to treat wrinkles and discoloration. More effective than superficial and micro peels, but less effective than deep peels.

Medium peel: *Same as* Medium chemical peel.

Melasma: A type of hyperpigmentation with a "dirty" appearance and irregular borders. An area of dark, blotchy skin that may develop on the face or neck during pregnancy or while using oral contraceptives.

Membranes: *Same as* Mucosa.

Mentoplasty: *Same as* Chin augmentation.

Micro peel: Application of a mild chemical, usually glycolic acid, to your skin. More effective than skin care alone, but less effective than a superficial peel.

Micro-pigmentation: *Same as* Cosmetic tattooing.

Mid-face-lift: *Same as* Cheek lift.

Milia: Skin eruptions that appear as tiny whiteheads. May occur along suture lines following eyelid surgery or throughout areas treated with deep chemical peels or laser. May either improve on their own or require further treatment.

Ml: Abbreviation for milliliter, which is a metric measure for fluid volume. (One pint is roughly equal to 500 ml. One ounce is equal to 30 ml.)

Mucosa: The lining on the inside of your nose or mouth. (Some doctors refer to mucosa as "the membranes.")

Nasal dorsum: The roof or backbone of the nose. Also called the dorsum of the nose.

Nasal septum: *Same as* Septum.

Nasolabial fold: The skin fold extending from the side of each nostril around the corner of the mouth, down toward the chin. Present with aging and formed by sagging cheeks. Usually improved by a face-lift.

Nose job: *Same as* Rhinoplasty.

Operating room fee: *Same as* Facility fee.

Outer thigh and buttock lift: Removes excess skin in the buttock and outer thigh region, resulting in tightening and lifting of the remaining skin.

Outpatient surgery: Allows the patient to return home the same day. Also known as day surgery or ambulatory surgery.

Panniculectomy: An operation to remove skin and fat from the lower abdomen, without tightening the fascia. Typically performed on previously obese people with back pain or hygiene problems related to extremely droopy abdominal skin.

Parrot beak: Also known as polly beak. A nasal deformity in which fullness above the tip of the nose causes the tip to lose its distinction from the dorsum of the nose.

Pectoralis muscle: The muscle between the ribs and the breast.

Phenol peel: *See* Deep chemical peel.

Photoaging: Accelerated skin aging that results from the cumulative effects of unprotected exposure to ultraviolet radiation from the sun and tanning beds.

Pixie ear: *Same as* Attached earlobe.

Plastic surgery: A broad surgical specialty that includes both reconstructive surgery and cosmetic surgery.

Platysma: A broad thin neck muscle that may become prominent with aging.

Platysmal bands: Cords of the platysma muscle that form with aging, extending from the jaw to the collarbone. May create a turkey gobbler appearance if severe.

Platysmaplasty: An operation to tighten the two platysma muscles by sewing them together in front of the neck, creating one continuous muscle instead of a pair of prominent bands.

Polyethylene: A plastic material used for facial implants. Resembles sea coral.

Preoperative testing: The required x-rays, EKG, and blood tests a few days prior to surgery. May be performed at a hospital or surgery facility.

Price: *See fees.*

Procerus muscles: Muscles which, together with the corrugators, make the vertical frown lines between the eyebrows.

Proplast: A plastic implant material similar to chewing gum. Formerly popular for facial augmentation. Withdrawn from the market after causing many complications.

Prosthetic material: Any material implanted into the body that is not derived from the body. May be synthetically made, such as plastic polymer, or naturally occuring, such as cadaver bone.

Ptosis: The medical term for droop. Pronounced *toe-sis*. (*Brow ptosis* refers to droopy eyebrows, and *breast ptosis* refers to droopy breasts.)

Pug nose: An upturned nose that is unattractive and unnatural.

Reconstructive surgery: The treatment of patients due to accidents, cancer, burns, birth defects, or other problems.

Rectus muscles: Abdominal muscles, also called abs.

Retin-A: A prescription topical cream that stimulates circulation to the skin, facilitates skin cell growth and turnover, thickens the deep layers of skin, and leads to a brighter, healthier complexion with smoother texture. Also called retinoic acid or tretinoin. Derived from vitamin A.

Revision surgery: Repeat surgery on the same part of the body, either to further improve the result or to correct a deformity.

Rhinoplasty: Cosmetic nasal surgery. The word is derived from the Greek terms *rhino* meaning nose and *plasty* meaning to shape or reform.

Rhytidectomy: *Same as* face-lift.

Rippling: A visible phenomenon that may follow breast augmentation. Small waves of liquid within the implant are transmitted to the skin of the breast, causing it to wrinkle or ripple.

Rosacea: A skin disorder in which the cheeks, nose, and chin become easily flushed in response to spicy foods, alcohol, or stress. Acne and spider veins may also develop.

Saddle bags: The fat deposits of the outer thighs.

Saline: Water with dissolved salt in the same concentration as it exists in the human body.

Saline breast implants: Breast implants filled with saline. Similar to water balloons. Made of a durable, pliable, plastic material called solid silicone.

Sclera: The white part of the eyeball.

Scleral show: Unnatural-looking result of lower eyelid retraction, which exposes the sclera below the pupil. May cause dry eye syndrome.

Sclerotherapy: Injecting a liquid chemical through a tiny needle directly into spider veins, causing them to contract and collapse.

Scowl lines: Furrows and vertical wrinkles between the eyebrows that give an angry appearance.

Sedation anesthesia: Also called twilight anesthesia or monitored anesthesia care (MAC). Uses intravenous medication to induce drowsiness and relaxation.

Septoplasty: Surgical modification of the septum of the nose with the goal to straighten it and improve breathing.

Septum: The wall inside the nose that separates the right and left nasal passages.

Seroma: A collection of clear fluid that weeps into the surgical site, under the skin, following surgery. (Your surgeon can remove most seromas with a needle in the office.)

Silastic: A solid plastic that may be white or clear, and pliable or stiff. May be used for facial augmentation.

Silicone gel: Jellylike silicone that has been used in some breast implants.

Silicone gel breast implants: Breast implants filled with liquid silicone gel. Withdrawn from the U.S. market in 1992. Expected to be available again in the future.

Sinusitis: Sinus infection. Usually due to internal nasal swelling if it occurs following rhinoplasty. Symptoms include foul nasal drainage, facial pain, headaches, and fevers. (If you have any of these symptoms, contact your plastic surgeon immediately.)

Skin care: A home-based program designed to decrease roughness, brighten complexion, minimize pore size, reduce blotches, and provide a healthier overall appearance.

Skin death: A complication of surgery that may occur where the skin is under tension or its blood supply is poor. May follow infection or hematoma. Most common in smokers.

Skin fold wrinkles: Wrinkles that develop around the nose and mouth as the cheeks sag with age. May be treated by face-lift.

SMAS: Stands for *s*ubcutaneous *musculo-a*poneurotic *s*ubstance. The layer of fibrous tissue under the facial skin, lifted and tightened during some types of face-lift.

Smile lines: *See* Dynamic wrinkles.

SPF: *Same as* Sun protection factor.

Spider veins: Tiny blood vessels that form within the skin, typically on the legs and face.

Steroids: Hormones given to patients orally or intravenously to reduce swelling and give a psychological lift following surgery.

Stretch mark: A tear in the deep layer of skin, resulting in a thinned, streaky appearance.

Subglandular: Describes where a breast implant can be placed—under the breast, which is a type of gland.

Submental fat: Fat under the chin.

Submuscular: Describes where a breast implant can be placed—under the pectoralis muscle.

Subpectoral: *See* Submuscular.

Subperiosteal face-lift: The deepest possible face-lift, in which all tissues are separated from the underlying bone and moved higher.

Suction lipectomy: *Same as* Liposuction.

Sun protection factor (SPF): The degree of a sun block's strength; the higher a product's number, the better it protects skin from harmful ultraviolet light.

Superficial chemical peel: A very controlled, mild injury to the skin from applying a chemical such as salicylic acid to treat wrinkles. More effective than micro peels, but less effective than medium peels.

Superficial peel: *Same as* Superficial chemical peel.

Surgeon's fee: The amount you pay your surgeon to perform a procedure. (The average surgeon's fee listed in each chapter was derived from a poll of plastic surgeons across the country. Cosmetic fees are similar throughout most of the country with the exception of the New York area, where they are consistently about 50 percent higher.)

Symmastia: The merging of the breasts into an indistinct mass. Occurs when the skin between them loses its attachment to the breastbone during surgery.

TCA (trichloroacetic acid): The chemical most commonly used for medium peels.

Telangiectasias: *Same as* Spider veins.

Telltale sign: A physical clue to the fact that someone had cosmetic surgery. Looks unnatural; can only be due to previous cosmetic surgery.

Textured breast implants: Implants' surface feels like dull sandpaper rather than being smooth.

Thigh-lift: *See* Inner thigh lift and Outer thigh lift.

Total body lift: Includes tummy tuck, inner thigh lift, and outer thigh and buttock lift.

Traditional liposuction: The original method of liposuction. Suctions out fat deposits through a thin tube, after stiffening the fat layer via tumescent fluid.

TRAM: *t*ransverse *r*ectus *a*bdominis *m*yocutaneous flap. A way to restore a breast following mastectomy by moving abdominal skin and fat. An extensive operation—not advised for breast augmentation.

Transaxillary breast augmentation: Placement of breast implants through an incision in the underarm. (Since the advent of the endoscope, this approach has regained popularity.)

Transconjunctival incision: An incision on the inside of the lower eyelid, sometimes used to remove fat from eyelids when skin removal is not necessary.

Transumbilical breast augmentation: Places breast implants through an incision in the belly button. Leads to an increased risk of intraoperative and postoperative problems due to the surgeon's restricted view during the procedure.

Tumescent fluid: Infused into fat prior to liposuction, making the fat stiff and therefore easier to suction. A mixture of saline, lidocaine, and adrenaline.

Tummy tuck: Surgery that removes excess abdominal skin and fat and tightens underlying fascia.

Twilight anesthesia: *Same as* Sedation anesthesia.

Ultralight chemical peel: *Same as* Micro peel.

Ultrasonic liposuction (UL): Combines the application of high-frequency sound waves with gentle suctioning.

Upper eyelid retraction: Inability to fully close the upper eyelid. Usually due to overzealous skin removal during eyelid surgery.

Varicose veins: Large distended veins beneath the skin. May appear as bluish bumps on the skin.

Witch's chin: Droopy chin skin after chin surgery has disrupted the attachments between skin and bone.

Wrinkle filler: Substance, such as collagen or fat, which is injected into the skin under each wrinkle. Pushes the depressed wrinkles outward and makes them less visible.

Wrinkle laser: *See* Laser resurfacing

Wrinkles: Linear depressions in the skin. Classified according to their cause as either crepe paper, dynamic, or skin fold wrinkles.

Bibliography

American Society of Plastic and Reconstructive Surgeons. *Plastic Surgery Procedural Statistics.* Arlington Heights, IL, 1999.

Musculosketal Transplant Foundation. *Musculosketal Transplant Foundation Patient Brochure.* Edison, NJ, 1999.

Nash, Joyce D. *What Your Doctor Can't Tell You About Cosmetic Surgery.* Oakland: New Harbinger Publications, 1995.

U.S. House Committee on Small Business. Subcommittee on Regulation, Business Opportunities, and Energy. *Unqualified Doctors Performing Cosmetic Surgery: Policies and Enforcement Activities of the Federal Trade Commission–Part I.* 101st Congress, first session, 4 April 1989.

U.S. House Committee on Small Business. Subcommittee on Regulation, Business Opportunities, and Energy. *Unqualified Doctors Performing Cosmetic Surgery: Policies and Enforcement Activities of the Federal Trade Commission–Part II.* 101st Congress, second session, 31 May 1989.

U.S. House Committee on Small Business. Subcommittee on Regulation, Business Opportunities, and Energy. *Cosmetic Surgery Procedures: Standards, Quality, and Certification of Nonhospital Operating Rooms–Part III.* 101st Congress, third session, 28 June 1989.

Index